Rob

To an.

stands overcoming) + new
beginnings, we are grateful
for you!

With Respect,

Cherise + Gordon Lilley

ENDORSEMENTS

"I have struggled with chronic pain for years, and this is the ONLY book I have read that genuinely helps. It's not another theology of suffering, but instead, it's REAL HOPE! It's inspiring, life-changing, practical, and liberating! It's rest for the soul; a word to the weary; and, a grace-filled ocean of spiritual healing! Words are never enough, but somehow these GOD-inspired words of wisdom, heart, and experience are. Get set free today!"

GREG OUTLAW, CEO, *All About God Ministries*

"This narrative is an incredible journey of courage, strength, endurance, and perseverance. One that will empower you to press on during your season of pain, distress, and hopelessness – to have the faith to believe God, trust Jesus for His unfailing presence, and the assurance of the Holy Spirit who will remind you of God's truth. 'He makes all things beautiful in His time.'"

DAVID PACKIAM, Chaplain, *Springs Rescue Mission*

"Gordon and Cherise are bringing hope to the hopeless, encouragement to the weary, and healing to the soul. Dive into this painful yet promising journey and be blessed by truth from their excerpts from the Word of God. The experience of these two people who have not only been there in suffering, but also, they continue to thrive there today."

MARK HEFFENTRAGER,
Director of Eagle Lake Camps, The Navigators

"Is chronic pain your daily companion? Chronic pain is complicated and impacts every aspect of life, as Gordon and Cherise Selley know. Their suffering has become the catalyst for their deep faith in Christ. In this book, the Selleys share how they have found freedom from 'the strangling arms of pain.' Readers can learn to taste opportunity and hope."

SUES HESS, Exec. Dir., Restore Innocence

PURSUE REAL
HOPE

DISCOVER BETTER LIVING
DESPITE YOUR PAIN

GORDON & CHERISE SELLEY

PURSUE REAL HOPE: Discover Better Living *Despite* Your Pain

Distributed globally by Boss Media.
New York | Los Angeles | London | Sydney

Paperback ISBN: 978-1-63337-497-3
Hardback ISBN: 978-1-63337-501-7
E-book ISBN: 978-1-63337-498-0
Library of Congress Control Number: 2021907646

Manufactured and printed in the United States of America

DEDICATION

To the lost voices of the millions who chronically suffer,
your cries are heard.

To our beautiful grandchildren, JJ and Harmony-Jae,
we love both of you immensely. The joy that you bring us has
lingered throughout this book project.

To God, for the realities of life and Your love.

CONTENTS

INTRODUCTION
BY CHERISE SELLEY

I STOOD AT THE DOORWAY of my husband's hospital room and stared at him. In all sincerity, I didn't know how to react. I desperately wanted to be the kind of wife who could bring our family through any crisis.

But this occasion was far beyond my life experience; it tested every part of who I was. Quite frankly, panic set in as my heart seemed to explode out of my chest. I stood motionless in deep shock. While observing what was happening in the hospital room, I hated watching the out-and-out destruction that pain was causing as our lives crumbled right before my eyes.

Gordon, my husband, was fighting for his life. His body glistened with profuse sweat, and his breathing resembled a pregnant woman during the height of labor. With each breath he took, his neck and chest muscles drew into spasms as deep moans bellowed from within his soul.

No, this wasn't the beginning of romantic bliss that newly-weds typically get to experience. Instead, this was the beginning of the end as we knew it, for this acute pain rudely intruded upon our young marriage at the six-month mark.

Sure, Gordon had pain for a few years before I ever met him, but it seemed like his history of painful battles were somewhat under control. Up until now, his pain remained neat and tidy, if there was such a thing, until the raging monster of tortuous suffering unleashed its fury upon him.

For hours, I listened to Gordon cry out for mercy as he barely coped with cascading bouts of burning, excessive pain. As insufferable as his fiery affliction was for him to bear, it had the same effect on me.

I couldn't take it any longer. My insides were riddling with nausea. Finding myself unable to watch this version of torture on the man I deeply loved, I scampered out of the room into the corner section of the waiting area.

While sitting alone, balled up in a fetal position, and staring out the window, the anesthesiologist specializing in pain management met me for a sober face-to-face meeting.

Initially, the doctor was trying to act clinically objective, describing aspects of what Gordon was trying to endure. But as our conversation continued, the doctor got emotional as he let me know that he and his colleagues were highly doubtful that my husband would be able to live through the magnitude of this out-of-control pain syndrome.

However, we discussed various options for emergency treatments. As a last-ditch effort, the doctors wanted to implement sympathetic blockades throughout his spinal column regions. Essentially, this type of pain-reducing treatment would shut down his nervous system, rendering him a quadriplegic temporarily.

The hope was that the excessive pain might calm down in a week or so after the sympathetic blockades were removed.

When I returned to Gordon's room, he consented to have the doctors administer the sympathetic blockades into his spinal regions. Once they did, he was in the state of quadriplegia that allowed him to only turn his head from side to side.

Finally, after a few hours, the pain had subsided long enough for me to speak with him about all that was happening.

Gordon carefully described his painful ordeal, saying that it felt as if someone had lit a match and placed it against his skin. He said that his pain was unimaginably challenging to bear.

Later the next day, we finally met with the primary care doctor who diagnosed Gordon with the most aggressive form of CRPS (Complex Regional Pain Syndrome), formerly known as RSD (Reflex Sympathetic Dystrophy). In fact, the doctor had said that Gordon presented with the worst case he had ever seen. All of his nerves were firing off like a fireworks finale that simply wouldn't end.

Suddenly, our newly formed marriage, which I had thought we were going to build together, collided with the trauma we were facing. Nothing was ever going to be the same again. The idea that our two boys, ages seven and four respectively, might grow up without their dad and stepdad caused overwhelming grief and tears to flood my eyes.

I was twenty-three years old with little work experience. I kept wondering what we were going to do. How was I supposed to make it on this earth without him?

Plus, the mental and emotional anguish of watching him suffer dimmed the lights on any hope for a brighter future. I could identify with Jesus's suffering as He prayed alone in the Garden of Gethsemane: "Abba, Father, for You, all things are possible; remove this cup from Me; yet not what I will, but what You will" (Mark 14:36).

"What are we going to do?" I asked, trying my best to keep the desperation and fear out of my voice.

Gordon's answer to my question has stuck with me for the past twenty-four years. "Honey, we are going to praise God through this ordeal. Pain is not the final signature of our lives."

I'll admit I didn't exactly share his courageous attitude at the time. Instead, I felt more like Job's wife, screaming inside, "Why don't you curse God and die" (Job 2:9)?

Yet, Gordon did just as he said. He led by example of handling painful trials, such as those that far exceed our capabilities. Moment by moment, then day by day, he offered his broken body to God as the only sacrifice he had left. And God met him. After I drew closer to God, eventually, He came upon me and filled my place of brokenness with something entirely hopeful.

Pain was not anything we ever asked for, yet it has been like a treasure hunt in the ocean's depths as we dove inward for powerful, transformative answers. Consequently, we found many golden nuggets of wisdom and inspiration that continue to help us live beyond our chronic suffering, even today.

Despite the pain he faces daily, Gordon has been in remission from his worst battles against CRPS for twenty-three years. Now he contends every day through varying bouts of neuropathic pain from having four neck surgeries and several levels of cervical spinal stenosis. As a result, Gordon has also accrued a compromised immune system over the years. This compromise has undermined other internal systems, causing ongoing kidney stone problems and an autoimmune disease of rheumatoid arthritis.

But regardless, as much as the pain has caused permanent damage to some areas of our former lives, it has also been a catalyst to discover some new ways of living that God has always intended for us.

These new ways of creative living include integrating a richer faith into our present circumstances, counting on a confident hope that infectiously spreads love, compassion, and generosity to others, and practically living out an abundant lifestyle, regardless of the severe hardships along the path of life.

INWARD TEARS

You might assume that more spiritually centered or mature people are immune from having their lives wrecked by suffering. After all, it's easy to believe that some unique souls have a better grasp of who they are, a greater sense of connection to God and their deeper inner selves, as well as healthier relationships with the world around them. Some people appear protectively wrapped within God's loving cocoon, at least from a distance.

But our assumptions aren't always accurate or correct, especially in this case. Life-crushing trials can happen to anyone, regardless of our religious beliefs, how many prayers we pray, how much we give to charity, how healthy we are mentally and emotionally, and how well we conduct ourselves in the affairs of this present world.

When it rains, those water-filled clouds in the sky drench both the good and the bad. No one gets a "grace card" that promises an escape from the horrific trials of life.

All of us experience trials and tests. All of us have cried inward tears of self-pity and discouragement during difficult seasons of our lives. And all of us can break when life's trials grow too overwhelming.

We may wish it wasn't so, but pain is part of the developmental process we humans must go through in life. Suffering challenges us to grow but not always in the ways we plan or desire.

None of us would ever volunteer to step into the furnace of bodily suffering and affliction. But those of us who live daily in that furnace aren't helping ourselves if we imagine that we alone have been singled out for pain while others seem to slide by without a concern or a tear.

You no longer have to hide your deep traumas or unmet

expectations about life that loudly shout from the voices inside your head. This fiery suffering will help you find the purest part of your true self.

You now have a second chance to discover truth, purpose, life, and God. It's an opportunity to seek that "still transcendent voice" within you that might unexpectedly echo a heartfelt message of wholeness and healing.

There is no better time than now to have your inward tears wiped away.

YOUR LIFE IS MORE THAN PAIN

You might be thinking, *You don't understand my pain.* And you're right; we don't, and nor does anyone else.

None of us can entirely understand the pain that you're suffering. We can have empathy for you. Still, we're not living on the inside of your body to know exactly what you might be experiencing.

Gordon and I are called to encourage you and let you know that you are more than the sum of all your pain. You are so much more than what you're feeling right now, though broken pieces of your life are scattered everywhere. You are more beautiful on the inside than you might realize, even in the worst times of your misery and anguish.

Yet there is an ongoing battle for your life. Through the clouded lens of pain, it's hard to remember this truth—a life of love wins every single time.

The battle isn't won within this vulnerable flesh of ours. Instead, our weapons of warfare are found in the Holy Spirit within us. If we allow our minds to drift away from the Spirit and onto our thorny pains, then the battle is fought on the enemy's terms.

This book is a reminder to move your painful battles to the battlefield where the Holy Spirit resides—that place that's located deep within your soul. Then your fight can happen on the advantageous conditions that Jesus Christ has set forth for you.

The battle then becomes His. You'll begin to notice how the truth will eventually rise to the surface, delivering you this fact: your pain belongs to God, and it is not yours always to keep.

LET'S GET STARTED

Perhaps this book has spoken to you because chronic pain is intricately woven into the fabric of your life.

If you're observing your loved one in pain or if you're the one who is enduring horrific pain, there is real hope that awaits you. Pursue it!

Gordon and I are grateful to share some of the deep treasures that we have uncovered throughout our pain-filled journey, ranging from Gordon's physical suffering to my emotional wreckage. We discovered that there are real, practical answers about your chronic suffering hidden within the mysteries of your faith.

You are not alone in your search for help.

Let's dive into the waters to find real treasures of hope for you today!

FALLING INTO
THE PAIN PIT

ACCORDING TO CLINICAL DEFINITIONS, chronic pain persists for three to six months, long past the time required to heal from a particular ailment. However, your original injury or illness seems to last, even after you were predicted to recover. Your nervous system continues to transmit pain signals throughout your body actively.

But clinical definitions only go so far. What's it like to live with chronic pain?

It can happen suddenly. The dream of the good life you sought to enjoy is turning into a nightmare as you fall over the ledge and into a dark, bottomless, and inescapable pit of pain and anguish.

This pain pit is a place of seemingly unloving darkness and isolation. It's a place where your freedoms give way to shackles. It's a place where hope for a better pain-free tomorrow seems lost. It's a place of complete isolation from those you loved and thought you knew.

PAIN CAN STRAIN OR BREAK RELATIONSHIPS

Living with chronic suffering can be a hideous experience. It's terrible when your broken body is waging war within you and against you.

Normal, healthy people find it difficult to sympathize with our life in the pit of pain because that's not where they live. But we must also admit that we create distance from them too, often relying on weak excuses to avoid spending time with them when we can't crawl out of the pain that seeks to define us.

We want to connect with others more deeply, sometimes desperately so, but we don't think we can stand the pain we'll experience in the effort. This tension can set up a mental tug-of-war—can we venture out to connect with others, or must we remain isolated in the pain pit?

Few people seem to grasp that sometimes, we can't communicate clearly with others. We face challenges that most people don't encounter when it comes to the simplest of social commitments: going to work, seeing others for dinner, attending church, or doing easy tasks.

Our social behaviors lead some to conclude that we are carelessly disregarding some of the essential things of life with others. They're convinced we choose to remain aloof and that we want to avoid creating stable relationships. They're not aware that we're finding it difficult to navigate the world of painful suffering successfully.

Society frequently misunderstands our suffering. Those of us who can't help revealing our pain may experience ostracism and exclusion. For instance, if we rely on canes, walkers, or other assistive devices to get around, we may arouse people's sympathy, evoke their disdain, or earn their impatience and displeasure for merely being in their way.

When we breathe with the help of an oxygen tank, wear prosthetic devices, demonstrate slurred speech, or can't stop our body from coiling up in pain as a result of severe neurological lesions, we may evoke stares and social distancing measures from those who can't see the beautiful human beings behind the pain.

Unbeknownst to those who are fine, millions of members in the chronic pain population don't use equipment or present with outward signs that reveal they're in some type of distress. They appear reasonably healthy, so they escape our notice. It's only when we listen to their stories that we learn how pain adversely affects their lives.

Even though they suffer, only their closest companions understand the true extent of their disability or how their undetectable pain is debilitating. People expect them to carry out all the typical daily activities that healthy people enjoy, but often they can't rise to the challenge.

While we're doing everything we can to deflect the hostile stares that others send our way, we must also confront our negative, self-destructive attitudes about our situation. Some of us may be tempted to deny the oppression we experience in the pain pit, but living in denial is no way to have a balanced, faithful life.

When we first fall into the pain pit, we know that we hurt tremendously—physically, mentally, and emotionally. Often, we hurt spiritually too. The beliefs and practices that once gave us joy may now seem lifeless and flatlined.

Once we've been in the pain pit for a while, even our closest family members, loved ones, and friends may become sources of additional pain. Some judge us for our aberrant behavior. Others may not feel our pain, but they sure can feel their pain, including how they think we have rejected them.

We may conclude that other people's lack of understanding and compassion have deeply wounded us in response.

This vicious cycle of negativity and recrimination makes it even more challenging to forgive each other, love each other, and build the deep relationships that make life worth living.

As we live in the pain pit, we may experience the loneliness of isolation. We may also have a tiny amount of hope for reconciling and connecting with others. But the one relationship we know we will experience firsthand is our relationship to our own physical and psychological pain.

FALLING FROM YOUR PREVIOUS LIFE

Once upon a time, you may have lived life with relative ease, making choices about your future without fear. Not anymore. You've undergone a dramatic and sudden fall from your previous state to your current life. You are not the person you were before. You're now facing a new normal. All bets are off.

You may feel like you're now living in some lowly and despised leper colony alongside fellow untouchables and undesirables. You may feel like you've taken up permanent residence among "the least of these." That's how Jesus described those who were hungry, thirsty, naked, or sick. Those who were strangers. Those who were prisoners. He had a special love for these suffering souls.

No matter what you call it, you never wanted to wind up here. You dug in your heels, fighting against this assignment with all your might. But you fell anyway, and here you are. Even though you've repeatedly stomped your heels on the bottom of your dirt-filled pit, demanding to be set free, you remain here regardless, stuck and isolated.

It's no surprise that in your frustration, you may give in to the unhealthy behaviors or thought patterns you've previously resisted. You may allow yourself to stew over feelings of anger and bitterness from your past. You may curse up a storm or cry oceans of tears, but these responses don't offer any consolation. In fact, they may even worsen your agitation.

You now know what it's like to have everything of value stripped from your life, such as your joy, your independence, and a good measure of your dignity. You sense you may be headed for an uncertain future of limited choices, none of them good.

Your social world may evaporate in the darkness of the pit. Only a few new friends are willing to connect with you on a deeper level in your current state.

There are many potential targets you could blame for your fate. You could blame others. You could blame God. Some people spend a lot of time and energy blaming both.

Nonetheless, the blame game won't help you recover from your fall into the pit.

A DOOR CALLED HOPE

Your pain pit can become a living hell if you make it into a place where you endlessly wage an all-out battle against your enemies, real or perceived, inside or outside yourself.

But you can transform your pit into a place of learning, growth, healing, forgiveness, and redemption if you're willing to wrestle with yourself about the predicament you face and take full responsibility for your decisions in life thus far.

It's in times of total honesty and vulnerability with ourselves and with God that our eyes become open to new possibilities for life in this dingy and dirty place. Whereas before, our focus had been on stewing, fuming, and doing battle with ourselves, we can now see doors we had never noticed beforehand that are opened to reveal the doorways of hope, opportunity, healing, and wholeness.

What will you do? Will you walk through the doors of opportunity and hope if God places these entryways onto your path? Can you still hope for a better tomorrow, or are you pass the point where you're willing to risk hope?

We've all seen what can happen when a person turns down all offers of help and hope, insisting, "I alone must figure this out. I alone can fix this."

The got-it-alone approach commonly brings further destruction, which can take various forms. New compulsive habits can be developed, such as taking on new addictions—food, opioids, or frivolously spending money—that tear apart relationships, destroy marriages, and break up families.

But we're not condemned to live a life of despair and self-destruction. Even if we're stuck in a dreaded hole in the ground, we still have life. Hope again arises when we begin to see the suffering Christ within us.

Even if we can't climb out of the pain pit or avoid many trials, we can walk through the fire to a better life. Even if we walk through life with a limp, we still can move ourselves forward—an inch or a mile—on the road of redemption.

Anymore stomping on the bottom of the pain pit can symbolize something unequivocally different than extreme anguish. You can now stomp on the head of the enemy, and you can figuratively trample on the gates of hell against your life. The power of this type of stomping will free you from your temporary painful suffering, bringing you into authority over this world's shackles.

Isn't that better than letting the fear of the unknown paralyze you from imagining and pursuing something better?

When you've landed at the very bottom of the pain pit of chronic suffering, you've finally found your ground floor on which to build your new life. There's no better time to reach out in faith to God, who is greater than any darkness, near or far.

Doors of opportunity and hope genuinely exists.

Can you see them?

Let's walk through these doors together by faith in the hopes of learning all we can about the causes of our suffering and the sources of our healing.

YOU ARE NOT ALONE

YOU'VE LANDED IN A PARADOX. You are alone, but you're not alone. Though pain makes you think you're isolated, you are not all by yourself to deal with your massive health debacle. The fact is that 50 million American adults struggle with chronic pain.

The Centers for Disease Control and Prevention says that one in five Americans experience chronic pain. In other words, 20 percent of us have seen our lives diminished by at least one of these unwelcome realities:

- Regular medical care
- Restrictions in mobility and daily activities
- Dependence on opioids
- Anxiety and depression
- Reduced quality of life

Other groups argue that the CDC's 50-million number is way too low. One group says that 70 million Americans suffer from chronic pain. Using a different model, another group claims chronic pain afflicts 116 million Americans—more than half of American adults.

Welcome to the paradox of chronic pain today. You are alone, but you're not alone! It can make you believe that no one in the world faces what you're facing. However, you're far from alone when trying to deal with your particular version of painful suffering.

Chronic pain sufferers come in all shapes and sizes. Many might look just like you. On the outside, they might resemble someone who appears to be completely healthy. But on the inside, you don't know how many people earnestly struggle throughout each day.

Though the medical statistics provide the big picture narrative about chronic pain, the real-life stories of those who suffer chronically are intensely personal. The ongoing pain cycles force you to deeply "feel" your afflictions and its unspeakable awfulness. When pain erupts again and again, and each time with more fury, how can you not take it personally?

It is on you, and it is in you. You are the one who has the out-of-breath, throbbing pain and who inwardly cries rivers of sorrowful tears. You are dealing with a shattered soul, for which you experience the brute realities of brokenness and are more lost than ever in a world that never seems to slow down. The aloneness makes you wonder if you can make it through another day.

Of course, your story is very personal. You're the one who senses and feels the deep hurts so that it seems as if everyone else has removed you from the relevant parts about living. And love? How do you muster the compassion within yourself to love others, especially when you believe that there is no compassion extended to you when you need it the most?

Chronic pain also does a number on your psyche, making you believe you're worthless and life itself senseless, which is magnified if you haven't attached any purposeful meaning to it. Your experience then becomes a slow death as you vulnerably allow guilt to sliver through the open spaces of your mind. No longer does your pain attack your body, but it invades the deepest parts of who you are. This onslaught against your entire being darkens your outlook even deeper into that place of nothingness.

FINDING LIGHT INSIDE THE DARK

God does not want us to remain stuck deep within the pain pit of our misery. Jesus loudly sighed with anguish whenever He witnessed the weight of brokenness on the people of this world. He also responded to our painful wounds by committing His life to brokenness.

Jesus was no stranger to pain. His flesh was repeatedly ripped from His bones during His flogging, making Him look almost unrecognizable as a human being. As a result, His life became an offering for everyone's sin as well as for those who greatly suffer. God made His powerful nature into our living reality as He demonstrated His love for us on the cross so that we might find real life through Him.

Through the luminous light of love, God reveals Himself clearly to our lives amid the dark places of our afflictions. God does not see darkness as we do. Darkness does not blind His sight to the hidden things of pain, nor is God fearful like us when we sense danger or have lost complete control over our lives.

God is love; God is NOT pain. Even though it is hard for us to understand how God's love can somehow be intertwined with suffering, we typically relate to the assumption that pain may feel like the closest thing we can relate to as evil. However, in the context of long-suffering, afflicting trials are not evil. Instead, these fiery tests for our lives become an integral part of our spiritual growth.

Pain isn't necessarily our enemy. For example, if we didn't have an alarm system for our bodies against harm, we wouldn't know how to take our hand off the hot burner of a stove. Furthermore, when the fire from the flames keeps burning even after we've quickly removed our fingers from the glowing coils, it's easy to believe in the realities of our torturous pain over anything else that's hopeful.

Emotions will not carry us through this hard place of affliction. Only the Spirit of God can fully overcome what seems like evil with good. He will make good out of our battles against painful trials, and from inside our deeper sufferings, grow us into the person we're becoming.

Although we feel alone, the truth delivers an opposite message from our emotions—we are not alone. Jesus Christ gave us a Helper after He ascended into the glorious heavens. He gave us the Holy Spirit, who resides on the inside of each of us who believes in Him. The Holy Spirit groans when we suffer the pangs of pain. He also wholly relates to our fears about the dark places in our minds. He lives there to guide us when we cannot see our way. He prays and comforts us during our times of grief-stricken despondency.

The Holy Spirit is real, and He is within us right now. We have to venture down the seemingly long path of faith with Him to discover that the road surprisingly contains endless miles of lessons about darkness and light.

SACRED PLACE OF TRANSFORMATION

Thomas Merton, one of the foremost spiritual thinkers of our time, wrote, "If we are only truly real 'in Him [referring to Jesus Christ],' it is because He shares His reality with us and makes it our own."

What we demand when we chronically suffer is a constant light in the darkness of our souls. We can't abandon the cross nor escape our painful trials to experience the life-giving presence of God.

We do not entirely give up our darkened journey because of this divine presence. The cross meant something altogether different for Jesus Christ than it does for us. For Him, it represented the heavy weight of sin and brokenness. For us, the empty cross is a symbol of ultimate hope. It also entails the gift we receive regarding our complete regenerative transformation.

It was God's way to become real for you in the darkness, knowing that He would eventually lift you from your struggles and place you on an expansive territory of freedom, light, and inner wholeness.

Once you relieve yourself from all of your self-doubting impulses in the dark, you'll clear the road of false debris and discover your true self as you walk out your faith more confidently. As a result, your obstacles will diminish behind your shadow, no matter the amount of obvious pain you're experiencing.

Those tight places of life will eventually open up. Your weaknesses turn out to be golden opportunities for God to demonstrate His power over what you thought were unattainable options for coping with chronic suffering.

Christ's power births new life, just as the caterpillar goes into a lonely cocoon until it transforms into a beautiful butterfly. From the old, you're becoming that new person while stationed within the enclosure of your darkness.

The solitude of the womb is where God created you. Assuredly, you remain among His most prized possessions, despite your feelings of horror and ugliness because of intractable pain.

Keep searching diligently for God in your place of darkness. Draw near to Him by faith, and He promises to draw near to you. And in doing so, God will generously free your heart from the chains of brokenness. Total anguish is not the final signature of your life.

God will become the light that shines brighter for you in your isolated world. The person you are probably most lonely for is the person you once were. The struggle is real. But the metamorphosis of the butterfly teaches you to become something new in that place of quarantine.

Let go of your former ways and your secret motives. There are no shortcuts to massive change. The process of transformation leaves nothing to waste. When your life becomes actualized by love, then your supernatural conversion suggests that the transcendent hand of God has touched you remarkably onto the starting line of your new reality.

Your place of loneliness forever turns into your sacred place of transformation.

You are alone, but you are not alone.

WALKING WITH A LIMP

THERE IS NO BETTER TIME THAN NOW to transform your life into something new, but the transformation process may feel more like wrestling with God since you've had unrelenting pain for so many years.

Through your long-suffering, your failure to fully embrace your painful circumstances is why you focus on your limp as you struggle to walk out your faith consistently. Thoughts regarding what others proclaim about the healing power of God seem hollow and upset you considerably—especially when nothing about your physical body shows significant improvement after all of your earnest requests.

Understandably, there is an authentic contradiction between how you try to believe in the power of your faith versus the silence of your prayers when healing doesn't come to cure your broken body.

Healing is allegedly available to all, but very few are healed from what you've witnessed. No wonder your walk of faith has a limp.

Your faith may be strong, but you know that belief in itself has not yet delivered a healing miracle. The whole concept can sometimes seem like a cruel joke. Very little inspires an attraction to God's love when you can hardly make it through your morning routine without having the pain remind you that today will be another tough one on your calendar.

It's the elephant in the room for you and for others who observe your unsuccessful chronic battles with pain. Your disbelief provides a lot of sadness, not only for you but also for everyone involved with your life.

Suffering is complicated. But do these complications define who you are in pain?

Can you expect sketchy results when it comes to healing from God? What if the purpose of healing goes far beyond your interpretations of getting total pain relief?

Many of us who experience barbaric pain fight these confounding questions daily. We wrestle with these thoughts of doubt, wondering if we're slipping backward in our faith. We do not want to become the person who develops a hardened heart, especially when we try to hold on to the one thing that keeps us together—our faith.

Nevertheless, when we focus on our limp, we tend to do what we do not want to do. We step backward in our faith. Our intention to walk in full belief becomes skewed with disbelief. Then we revert to what we can see, forsaking the power behind our faith of what is unseen to the average eye. We focus on getting rid of our pain totally so that we can walk without a limp. Yet healing involves so much more than the physical body.

God has not called you to get back to your old normal nor to recapture the lifestyle you once lived. He does not promise to revise your past, nor does He erase your failures or rid your body of pain. God doesn't put His new garment of transformation on top of your old. The old parts about you are not subject to lifetime therapy, but rather, they are already presumed to be dead. They died with Christ on the cross when you pledged your life to Him.

You now have the freedom to see your life differently as a new person, whether you have that awful limp or not, or whether you are still weak, broken, and somewhat useless.

Healing doesn't necessarily equate to living a pain-free life. On the contrary, healing is so much more than what we think we can control about having perfect health. While we yearn for total pain relief, our attention returns to our fleshly cravings regarding what we can see, feel, and interpret with our bodies and minds.

But what about the value of the parts we don't see every day, such as our spirits?

Tap into the new person of who you are, created by God. Put on the mindset of Christ, learn invaluable knowledge from the

Word, and let your prayers transform your entire being from who you were previously into who you're now becoming.

Healing is about wholeness. And wholeness encourages you to walk with a renewed and inspired purpose, though you may still limp along at a slower pace.

Through long-suffering, you're going to discover that healing fits squarely into wholeness, which is your gift of salvation from Christ. You're made whole through Christ's crucifixion that happened 2,000 years ago. Your wholeness helps to eliminate those thoughts of doubt and suspicion that rumble around in your head about who God is.

Because of chronic pain, many of us have a hard time fully grasping this concept of wholeness where an infinite God truly desires to connect with broken-down, finite persons like us. We might theoretically know the good news of Christ's gospel. Still, for some reason, we often dismiss this relevant union between God and ourselves because of our aggressively hurting bodies and our doubting minds.

Indeed, suffering can remain complicated, especially over the long-term. But don't let your pain destroy your faith or stand in the way of the connection that God desires to have with you. Let it lead your way to Him.

And when in the middle of chronic suffering, your journey becomes overwhelming, it's always prudent to get back to the basics of your faith.

Believe! But also seek healing for the seasons of unbelief!

ADVERSITY VS. SUFFERING

These two words may seem the same, but adversity differs significantly from suffering.

Adversity tends to be more temporary.

When faced with the adversity that comes at us from other people and factors beyond our control, many of us know how to rouse ourselves, pull ourselves up by our bootstraps, and attempt to overcome whatever challenges we're facing. We may be weak and weary, but our track record of successful past battles against adversity encourages us to temporarily put aside our weaknesses, gather our strength, and find the energy to overcome.

But when faced with profound suffering that arises up from within us, everything changes. Suddenly, you lack the energy and enthusiasm to overcome your physical torture. You struggle to summon your strength when your daily companion is utter weakness. Even the pleasurable experiences you once enjoyed are now robbed of their comfort due to your chronic, throbbing pain that never seems to let up.

It looks like the floor of your pain pit consists of deep, miry clay that traps you like quicksand the more you work to extricate yourself. Any dreams you may have about reconstructing your life and trying to live as fully as you once did bring only stinging heartache and unspeakable discouragement. You feel like you're running on empty with nothing left in the reserve tank but fumes.

Whereas adversity waxes and wanes, suffering is long-lasting. It will likely need to be endured for extended periods, requiring you to hang on for dear life against seemingly impossible odds. You may be able to overcome adversity with the force of your will, but prolonged suffering isn't a force you can conquer with your power.

Standing up to painful afflictions requires more than the intellectual concepts in your mind or your body's brute physical strength. These types of trials call for your response of faith and trust in someone much smarter and more durable than you.

DEEP TRANSFORMATION

"O, the Depth" is the title of a brilliant sermon by British pastor and prolific author T. Austin-Sparks. Its central theme is that suffering brings something of real value to our lives. Painful afflictions bring us face to face with extensive testing, and as stated earlier, it's at the bottom of our souls where real change starts to happen.

Deep-down suffering not only brings us up close and personal with our limitations, but it shows us that we can't power through with sheer mental energy or muscle strength. We need deep transformation, which only comes from God and His profound love for us.

This type of suffering takes you down to the murky depths of your being that has yet to be explored. It demands that you choose faith in God and trust in His revealed plans for your life. It opens your heart to receive the power of God's truth in Scripture, transforming your soul and replacing your old, broken self with your newly redeemed person.

Austin-Sparks reminded us that these trials, testing, and profound suffering often accompany God's essential and sovereign work in the lives of His people. His divine energy can empower the transformation going on within us. We need to trust Him, get out of His way, and let Him do His work.

We can't always see the profound changes going on, mainly because we're caught up in the rapid pace of life. But while we're living on the surface, God is at work on our seemingly lifeless parts. Slowly, but inevitably, His love overcomes our periods of hesitation, doubt, and blindness to the profound truth that is bubbling below. In time, we will see that who we are in pain opens our eyes in new ways to the vast depths of real power stored within us.

Austin-Sparks thought we should be thankful for the intense value that suffering brings to our lives. After all, people who aren't wracked by chronic pain rarely travel in these zones. However, suffering offers us entry into the incredible wonders of this hidden world and the inner regeneration that takes place there.

As Jesus showed in His parable of the sower that when seeds fall on the rocky soil, they have no deep roots and soon wither and die. When seeds grow in good soil, their roots reach down into the deeper layers of the earth. They produce bountiful crops, perhaps as much as 100 times the seed that was sown initially.

Through our unrelenting pain, God directs us away from the shallow soil of this world's pleasures to the richness of the deep soil of His eternal Kingdom, which is His rule, even over every DNA molecule of our individual being.

Nothing of real value ever comes cheap. Our inner transformation happens as we carry our crosses of suffering, which connect to the core of our pain and beyond, to the infinite parts of God's love and mercy.

SEEING YOUR LIMP FROM A DIFFERENT ANGLE

Who are you in pain?

Do you focus on your suffering? Or do you focus on the transformation that the pain brings about in you?

Do you focus on the things that your pain has taken from your life, or do you focus on how your pain has prepared you for a different life?

Do you focus on your limp, or do you focus on your particular walk of faith?

You're not doing yourself any favors if you continually dwell on how you limp when you walk or on the painful medical procedures you must undergo or on all that pain has taken from you.

The way you look at your limp comes to pass through different optics of single-focused reliance on hopefulness. Instead, try giving your attention to the path of faith you hope to walk courageously. God has promised to show you His grace, and you can see it if you focus your spiritual eyes on the profound changes that are happening deep inside of you.

From one angle, all you can see is your limp, a troubling sign of your weakness. But from another angle, you can see the power of God at work through your chronic suffering. You're getting a preview of the eternal you, the inner person no longer twisted and defined by your broken body.

God has disqualified you from the standard-issue good life or some version of the American dream. He has chosen you for something much higher. Your chronic suffering tests your faith and prepares you for an eternity in His Kingdom, limp and all.

Chances are, your limp may worsen as you age or as you develop other pain syndromes, which often happens to chronic pain sufferers with compromised immune systems. But declines in your physical prognosis don't limit your spiritual growth. That's why you shouldn't concentrate on your limp but on your spiritual journey.

At times, the journey can be a wrestling match as you pray to and argue with God. You can't injure God, nor will He punish you for your inquisitive nature. Your transformation demands your conscientious and complete participation in the process.

Then there will be times when the journey seems like a battle between light and darkness. The darkness sometimes appears to grow darker during your most profound bouts of suffering, but the glimpse of light you see can illuminate and drive away that darkness.

So, who are you in pain?

Short answer: you are who you choose to be!

"God does not give us overcoming life," said Oswald Chambers, the Scottish pastor and author of *My Utmost for His Highest*. "He gives us life as we overcome."

BE A BENEDICTION

"A benediction is a blessing to impart," said T. Austin-Sparks in another one of his excellent sermons. "And we ought to be a benediction. We ought to be God's real grace in this world, the blessing of God to others."

Can you impart a benediction of blessing upon others even as you wrestle in the depths of suffering?

That's the transformational point of God's grace. He takes the awful things, the wrecking balls in our lives, the dark forces that fight for our destruction, and transforms them into blessings.

The blessings you have experienced through suffering can now be a source of benefit for others. You may not realize it yet, but you are a walking, talking manifestation of the hope that defies all destruction and despair.

Hold on a little while longer. The blessing is coming. It does not arrive by the absence of pain. Instead, it comes from the steadfast walk through the very thing that you are trying to pray away, and ironically, that may not go away.

Even though your life appears disjointed, a beautiful flower has taken deep root within you. That flower will eventually bloom and burst forth, sharing the fragrance of God's remarkable power of transformation with everyone with whom you come into contact.

You can't force the flower to open, but if you trust God's grace, He will bring forth the fragrant, life-giving bloom.

WHEN YOU FEEL LIKE GIVING UP

MANY OF US WILL GO TO GREAT LENGTHS to secure any pain relief. Without even thinking twice, we will do almost anything and spend everything we have (or don't have) to make it go away.

Chronic suffering is a complicated beast. In the early onset of our affliction, the focus is to get rid of our pain. Then when this doesn't happen after six months, the mode of care changes dramatically. The focus is no longer on the total amelioration, or improvement, of our symptoms. Instead, the strategy adjusts into the management of our pain.

This untamed beast tends to grow larger over time, not only in power, but it also forcefully causes further destruction to every aspect of our lives. Consequently, we develop additional unforeseen symptoms that are separate from our original injuries. Compromised immune systems give birth to other frightening beasts of pain, such as:

- Rheumatoid arthritis
- Kidney stones
- Fibromyalgia
- Hypertension
- Chronic fatigue
- Severe bouts of depression

The list mentioned above is comprised of just a few diseases that are spawned by our chronic pain. The catalog of other pain syndromes is way too large to give here. Chronic pain runs wild throughout every system of our bodies and destroys any physical evidence to prove that we are qualified to pursue a meaningful life. This beast loves to rampage in the darkness of our minds. It tortures our thoughts. Chaos and fear feed this ugly creature as it tries to take captive and demolish every good impression we have about our future.

Our bodies try to resist this flesh-pounding pain. This ferocious creature doesn't care about what we want and our welfare. It mightily tries to destroy, steal, and devour us completely. Amid this ongoing battle, we eventually begin to slow down from the lingering effects of extreme fatigue. It's as if we knowingly realize that we're going to have to surrender to this brute's painful clutches anyway.

Does this mean that we are doomed to have this creature rule over the rest of our lives? The scariest thing to come to terms with is that we are likely trying to run away from ourselves in this state.

CAUGHT IN A VICIOUS LOOP

Our hope is to escape from the worst of suffering. Then we realize the inevitable, that our lives might turn out messier than we ever envisioned.

Though we've learned many lessons about the darkness and the light, we continue to find ourselves desperate for relief. We are tired of the unfair chase of pain against our lives.

What choices do we have left? On the one hand, our faith fuels us with inspiring power. On the other hand, painful suffering depletes every aspect of who we are, including our measure of faith. This vicious cycle continually repeats over and over as throbbing pain turns into chronic suffering that eventually turns into decades of unrelenting frustration and exhaustion.

Naturally, you do what you can to survive this nightmare. Your life enters into an unhealthy loop, chasing after your symptoms to do something about them. The longer the suffering nightmare lasts, the less you remember what it feels like to live a pain-free existence. Instead, you settle for trying to dull the worst of your pain.

You make some steps of forward movement and experience temporary relief, only to loop back into more considerable pain and suffering. Still, you somehow keep trying to tame this beast with every breath still left in your lungs.

You will drain the medical system's resources to try different combinations of prescriptions, undergo more rounds of therapeutic modalities, or volunteer for riskier surgeries. You may start thinking you're a guinea pig, but your desperation overrides your discernment about what to do next.

Notwithstanding, most of us will keep fighting, even if we feel powerless. If our faith feels powerless, we'll turn to unfamiliar methods to find that *one* antidote that may give us provisional relief. We will dabble with unheard-of healing alternatives, rub CBD creams all over our bodies, or submit ourselves to far-out fad diets. We will look under every rock to find the solutions to our pain.

Many of us find ourselves trapped within this loop, trying to cure our elusive symptoms while being overwhelmed with the actual agony of its ever-present reality.

So what do we do next during our battle against the beast of chronic pain?

And what if our giant-size illness is incurable?

LET'S GET REAL

Nothing around your physical existence speaks life, and seriously, no one else has to point out this observation to you. You have already died a thousand deaths since you were inflicted with your pain. No matter how you try to spin the facts, nothing is the same in your world.

This reality is indelibly imprinted upon your memories. Over and over again, no matter what you try or do, the same theme echoes throughout your thoughts: *Nothing will ever be the same.*

Deep down, you know that today, you're a shell of the person you used to be. You've forgotten what a pain-free existence means. If you did happen to experience it, you're still not sure how you would start again.

Broken pieces of your life lay all around you. Time kept passing you as the years piled up. What was once central to your purpose seems outdated. Your skills have been placed on a top shelf—a high, hard-to-reach section that seems perpetually out of reach.

But in reality, you're not pain-free. You've been drained of too much energy to imagine starting your life over again. Sadly, you know it's much more challenging, if not impossible, with this giant monster still hanging onto you. Everything is heavier. Every movement is slower. Bending over to smell the roses might cause you additional episodes of pain, too. Nothing seems to work out for you.

Frankly, it takes far-too-much effort to think positively, and exhaustion is the only gas left in your tank, not even allowing you to circle the block.

Let's get real. Thoughts of suicide have come into your mind hundreds, if not thousands of times over the years. Instead of experiencing the four seasons of life, it feels like you've experienced one long winter of icy gloom.

Why keep going?

What is left in this life for you if you have nothing more to give?

THE SHEEP AND THE SHEPHERD

Picture yourself as a sheep, safely inside your pen. All of your wild enemies are outside, clawing away to get inside with you. All you can see is the dripping saliva from their muscled jaws and their sharp teeth curled above their lips. All you can hear are their growls, and from their closeness behind the gate, you can smell their rancid breath.

There is a point of entry into your pen through the gate. This threshold desperately needs to be guarded. To prevent your enemy from entering, you attempt to lie down at the entryway to keep the gate firmly closed. Yet as sheep, you are the prey because you are not fully equipped to deal with the enemy's explosive strength as its brute force tries to gain entry.

What you need is a shepherd. You need one who is more capable than you to protect you. You need the kind of shepherd who will put everything on the line for you, even if it means to sacrifice Himself at the gate for your safety and benefit.

There is only one Good Shepherd. He has voluntarily, out of love for you, put Himself in harm's way for you.

Allow Jesus to become *that* gatekeeper in that rugged territory between your suicidal thoughts and you. He is the only one who can bear that kind of pressure and entirely understand your anguishing pain about life and death.

Jesus also offered His life so you wouldn't have to, even if it was for you alone. He is the one who exists forever to be in *that* space, knowing that you are unable to stand against the evil that lurks beyond the gates. Jesus is at the threshold, keeping that gate closed for your safekeeping.

Finally, we are the sheep who tend to blindly wander during times of intense trauma. Jesus is also the only one who can give meaning to those dangerous places of suffering for you as He calls you back to the fold.

MAKE A SMART CHOICE

Thoughts of suicide are bound to come when dealing with long-suffering, whether your seemingly intractable pain lasts for a year or decades. But is taking your life the right thing to do?

How do you continue to take your next breath and put your next step forward without giving up?

The power of truth shines its light regarding who we are and what we're purposed to do. Without a doubt, we've already experienced an overload of misery from chronic suffering.

Realistically, however, we'll probably die thousands of more deaths before the expiration of our lives. Though our hearts cry for the kind of hope that we think would best suit our needs, we will most likely have to deal with more physical pain, and concurrently, we'll have to swat away those destructive thoughts that propose we take the easy way out of this temporal world.

Make a smart choice to live! The response is *that* straightforward. Giving up is not part of the transformation process for human life.

Although our bodies, minds, and emotions have undergone rigid opposition and brutal contradiction, this doesn't mean that our crushed spirits have to yield to the temptations of death.

For the truth is that we already died with Christ. Therefore, our spirits live forever, regardless of our short stint during this developmental stage of life on Earth.

Trying to make the right choice about committing suicide presents far-more complexities than trying to cope with chronic suffering. For instance, are you confident about what lies beyond the boundaries of life as you know it?

Do you comprehend all of the mysteries of God about life and death?

And do you travel through galaxies of isolated darkness before seeing beams of glorious light?

These confounding ideas are simply the tip of the iceberg. There are considerably more unanswered questions about the afterlife that man cannot sufficiently reply to with absolute truth, at least not yet.

Besides, why interfere with God's eternal work in your life, transforming you into that new, reborn, repurposed person that He created you to be?

Do you grasp the intricacies of His transformation process to make your new life happen for you?

While love hasn't prevented your painful trials, it still guides you into the exposing reality of the kingdom of heaven, whether here and now or later down the road of your faith.

After a while, you'll face the deeper side of love down this path. You'll discover that love kills those vivid images that make you feel chased continuously by wild beasts.

Meanwhile, hang in there. Do not try to fight your invisible monsters with your bare hands. Instead, grab on to the Holy Spirit's power within you so that you can persevere through anything successfully.

Never forget that you are loved and preserved by the Good Shepherd, who is the gatekeeper of your soul.

SANDCASTLES WASHED AWAY

OUR BATTLES WITH CHRONIC PAIN break up the unhealthy parts of our fleshly nature. While this purification seems like an exercise of dying to ourselves, it also demonstrates God's creative process as He makes new life, which only He can see, sprout from the lifeless parts deep inside of us.

This new life begins to develop as we feel the pain pressing into our old lifestyles. Though we might believe we're undergoing complete ruin from our suffering, what's actually happening is that our trapped identity in God is being released for the purpose of freedom.

When the wind of freedom blows against your being, you'll begin to make the kind of choices that represent new living. This is when you can choose to look past the events of your painful afflictions.

The more you see past your pain, the more your spirit will recognize this new growth taking root down in the core of who you are.

Your newfound urges, no matter how tiny and subtle, will eventually open you up to fresh perspectives about experiencing an entirely new side of life. Believe it or not, this purification process begins with God's divine influence directly on the most vulnerable parts of your brokenness.

Your spirit—which is the deepest part of who you are—is being reformed by God in your suffering furnace. Rather than plead for your former life, your spirit now craves new life, precisely one that is free from the corruption of your mind in the flesh.

It's as if your life represents a sword that's been placed within a fiery crucible. When your blade is removed from the scalding flames, the blacksmith gently wipes off the dross from who you are. No longer is the old you alive, but instead, you've become a new, shining sword in the spirit, brilliantly reflecting God's regenerative creativity within you.

This birth of change that you're sensing is hard to fathom. For too long, you've lived with the feeling of utter loneliness, and now God is revealing to you a part of Himself. He doesn't want your loneliness. Instead, God wants to fulfill your deepest needs as you're experiencing the dawn of this whole-person fulfillment.

Your pain journey has already exposed you to supernatural experiences that you find hard to explain to yourself and to others who have been part of this unsteady expedition. God's inner work of purification can be equally difficult to understand or articulate.

Imagine if you've never seen a tree, but you came upon it for the first time. How would you explain the nature of a tree to someone else? While you know the truth of the tree's reality, you likely do not have the correct words to accurately describe its nature. The same principle applies to some of the groaning patterns that the Holy Spirit gives you for the first time. Often, these experiences are beyond words and difficult to explain.

Still, there are occasions when you can't resist describing these new promptings to others. Even though you can't always effectively convey what's going on inside you, God's internal nudges send you crystal-clear messages. God loves you. He desires to live fully within you. He is working within you to heal your wounds for His greater purposes. His mysterious ways encourage you to live with hopeful ideals rather than giving in to the shadows of your chronic suffering.

You are on an excursion of change. As with other travels, once the train leaves the station, new vistas appear. As the scenery changes, so does your mindset. The way you think about your painfully despicable circumstances will gradually, but inevitably, start to change as you travel farther and farther into a new way of living.

As your transformation expedition continues, you will see that one creative change within you leads to another and then another. Before you know it, you begin to think new thoughts, feel new feelings, and see the world in a new light. You may not always realize it, but God is at work within you, playing an integral role in reforming your deepest desires and yearnings.

Regardless, many of us will innately dismiss God's creative process because of our fears that suggest that we will not be capable of living a better life. We wonder if our thoughts are real or pretend. We've already endured hardship beyond belief, so we tend to shelve any other choices about better living. As a result, we remain risk-averse to any other lifestyle options that might be feasible.

However, being stuck is not a reasonable excuse for remaining stuck within a place we want to leave. Though we do not trust ourselves, this does not mean that we can't grow in trust of what God is doing within us.

Whatever our minds focus on will eventually grow. When we focus on the Holy Spirit's truth, then we can let go of those tightly gripped feelings of being stuck. Then through our increasing trust in God, we can allow these intimate urges to lead our approach to a new way of living.

Soon, you'll discover that these divine impulses stir the trust process between God and you. It provides the kind of hope that slowly intensifies as your mind begins to fixate on what's hopeful instead of what's despairing.

GOD'S CREATIVE WAYS

Being smashed down to nothing through painful suffering is comparable to waves along the coastline crashing mightily against the shore, representing God's overwhelming power.

When conditioned for years to live with chronic pain, it's hard to accept that those same powerful waves can also settle on the sandy shores so gently that it's as if a mother is rocking her precious child to sleep.

That's what part of the creative process entails—peaceful order arising from violent chaos. It's God's way to place His finger on our wills to encourage us to build our new houses on a solid foundation of wisdom. When His touch is heavy on our purpose, He's opening our eyes to the more profound meaning for which we're created.

Since we are finite and temporal, our lives are the finite shoreline next to God's infinite salt waters. We build sandcastles to decorate the shores, but they will last for a short while and then collapse back to its purest form whenever the waters pour over them. Then we disintegrate into a grain of sand that becomes molded again by Christ's mystifying inventiveness.

Not surprisingly, God isn't finite like us. We have tried to carve out beautiful sandcastles for our lives. We've attempted to build replicas of the best of what the world has to offer. But God operates differently, perpetually renewing our hearts as we are part of something much bigger than what we see of ourselves in this present reality.

When it seems like you're being knocked around by succeeding cycles of powerful, destructive waves, think of your life as a tiny grain of sand, a small part of the heavenly sandcastle God is building to last for all eternity.

A great mystery is revealed in the power of waves. God's redemptive energy tirelessly works to remold human lives, using suffering to transform our grains of sand into a beautiful, artistic creation.

A MIND-BOGGLING SPIRITUAL UNION

By bringing us in touch with God's Spirit, we are experiencing a new communion in our lives, which brings forth the life-giving ways of Jesus Christ into our being. The fusion between God and us is primarily spiritual, validating that we've joined into a permanent, spiritual union with Him.

While we can't summon how the waves should wash onto the shore, we can still be observers of this rhythmic cycle of life as we play our part in the fulfillment of God's ultimate purpose. We must remember to walk in faith, and before long, our faith-walk turns into a journey of sacred trust.

To trust God is to know Him so deeply that our wills become His. This mysterious process happens when we surrender to His creative work. We then have an exclusive union with God, which is a mind-blowing honor on every level. It will likely transcend our thoughts and understanding about spirituality while inspiring our future upwards on the wings of optimism and solidified hope.

The more you expose your actual being to God during your renovation from old to new, the more He floods your life with unequaled love and wisdom. Once you've had a taste of the deep communion with God, then your life's shallow surfaces will fail to satisfy your heart's desires.

Except for the sand itself, nothing that represents our lives lasts forever. The Holy Spirit makes our inner being immovable, even though the waves may be taking down the sandcastles of our fleshly lifestyle.

Why worry if the ocean waves wash away your sandcastles?

Do you recognize that you're beginning to fill up with the essence of a divine purpose?

INTO THE DEEP WATERS

Why venture out into the deep ocean when it seems so altogether safe in the shallow waters next to the shore?

Chronic pain's devastating power has caused you to operate with only half of your abilities. Consequently, there's an understandable tendency to stay safe and remain fearfully close to the beach. The idea of exploring the ocean's depths seems impractical or even dangerous, especially as you experience more pain eruptions.

Even though you are tempted to play it safe, there's a spark of inspiration calling you to venture out into deeper waters. You may feel comfortable in your protective physical and psychological bubble, but such comfort can become a trap that prevents you from experiencing your next stage of restoration.

You have a choice. You can either remain safe, living only on the surface of life, or dare to discover the depths beyond the boundary of your self-imposed limitations. You'll most likely have to choose the path of resistance to break the constraints of painful living.

So, how deep is deep? Picture this. The deepest known point in Earth's oceans is the Mariana Trench area that reaches down to 36,070 feet below sea level. If you were to turn Mount Everest upside down into the ocean, you would still need to go another mile further down to reach this vast oceanic trench's depths.

Most of this dark underwater world is too deep for humans to visit, so it remains mostly unexplored. But thanks to deep-sea robots and other technological tools, we know that unusual life forms exist in this unexpected place. Some of these creepy-looking creatures have developed unique body structures that have allowed them to adapt to the extreme pressures of living at such great depths.

Like the oceans, we have unexplored depths in our own lives. There is a vast ocean within us that reaches far beyond our chronic suffering. We may be afraid of finding "monsters" lurking there, but God dwells in these depths through His Spirit. If we never explore them, we will remain unaware of who we are and untouched by the love and grace that God has for us.

Are you willing to venture down into your unknown depths? If you are ready, you will find treasures you never knew existed, and your small world of pain can become a vast world of new life.

Many people allow caution or fear to prevent them from going deep, but you will encounter the Holy Spirit living within these parts of your inner person.

Do you recognize His voice when He speaks to you, or does His presence seem as unfamiliar as the freaky creatures living at the bottom of the ocean?

YOUR DEEP-SEA MAP

You do not need to pack a heavy bag in the pursuit of the deep. However, you're going to need God's Word inwardly on your journey. The Word of God centers on your ability to have vision when exploring your dormant parts. Importantly, you need to understand precisely what you're observing about yourself and your interpretation of what God is doing within you.

When navigating inwardly, it would be best to surrender to the truth and allow it to grapple with the parts of your humanity that dwells in the shadows of your soul.

God's Word supplies an illumination of truth to direct you into the darkest and scariest parts of who you are. It brings light to darkness, strips away the false images of yourself, and quiets the shrieking sounds of terror in your places of silence.

His Word is truth. It will enable you to see what you had overlooked that was in front of you all along—His transforming power during your times of painful trials and tribulation.

When you're experiencing chronic pain, it's mighty difficult to assume that the Word intends to straighten up your life. Your mind creates suppositions that carry a tone of harshness and shame, especially if you have experienced unrelenting pain for quite some time. You, or others, hint that something in your life must be causing your long-term suffering, that somehow you are part of the problem.

The process of healing seems juxtaposed from how you might interpret God's powerful love for your life. It's as though the Word is scolding you into righteousness. Regarding God's promises of healing for all your brokenness, this assurance seems unlikely. It carries a religious contingency that perhaps some of your circumstances might work out for your benefit, only if you become part of the solution.

Can you sense the wagging of a religious finger of judgment over your life?

You do the work. You submit to God. You must read His Word to get the right answers to solve your miserable failures.

The main point of the Word becomes lost in the translation when guilt and shame reverberate throughout the message. We know that shame is not part of Jesus's gospel whatsoever. However, when someone else forces you to become the determining factor of "getting right with God," then you're missing the whole point about what lies in the deepest part of your being.

Jesus Christ, the Holy Spirit, and God the Father strongly contradict the feelings of shame as you carry a painful cross of brokenness throughout this life. This factual truth is found in the Word of God.

Shame makes you feel utterly powerless over your life's circumstances. On the contrary, God's Word inspires an overcoming spirit within you, bringing an uplifting power of faith that transcends any guilt and shame.

God's outcome to everything is love, and we can be assured through His Word that love conquers all.

Open a Bible, crack the gilding, turn the pages, and find those verses to see what God wants to reveal to you. You'll discover that His message of truth is redemption, not condemnation, and salvation, not incompleteness, eternal life, not an experience of having a shameful death.

Keep your Bible close to your heart. Read and study it as it will spiritually construct new eyes for you to see and new ears for you to hear the Holy Spirit in your places of the deep.

The more you surrender all your parts to God through His Word, the more you will experience the vitalizing aspects of His Spirit. As a result, you're going to gain the extra strength of the Holy Spirit to carry you onward throughout these challenging times.

No longer will your discouragements override this recently developed vision you have after discovering the new life you can now share with God.

NO MORE DOUBTS

HOPE BRINGS INSPIRATION to us on our journeys of life.

However, your experience might not seem very inspiring. You might be so dehydrated from losing hope that you can't even detect how thirsty you are from not receiving the proper nourishment of what authentic hope offers.

If hope is something unconquerable by this world's painful adversities, then why do so many people eventually lose it?

We tend to rely on the successful outcomes that hope may bring into our lives. Yet, the confidence we receive from it slips from our fingertips when we demand too much of it. When one positive thing happens on our behalf, we believe other hopeful possibilities may also exist for us, especially those things we lack in our lives, such as if you are:

- *Struggling with a severe illness or painful disease, you probably hope for better health.*
- *Holding on to your last penny before going bankrupt, you likely hope for more money.*
- *Living a dangerously chaotic lifestyle, you longingly hope for safety and peaceful solitude.*
- *Feeling lonely, then you eagerly hope for loving companionship.*

The list is lengthy for what we expect hope to deliver to us. It's easy to fall into the trap and assume that it will guarantee that a majority of our wishes will somehow come true. When we begin to believe in our wish list, it's easy to think that our passionate desires now equate to our basic living needs.

We expect our lofty wishes to produce tangible results, to bring miraculous solutions to our many needs, which become the essentials of our lives. Then when these essential needs are not satisfactorily met, we become crushed by disappointment and despair.

Further emotional damage occurs when we accumulate a mountain of unmet expectations in our hearts, mostly when our chronic pain does not disappear. Of course, painful suffering rears its ugly head again during the most inconvenient times to create more and more unmet expectations. Putting our hope into wish lists is no different than putting our faith into useless idols. There is no power in our wish lists, nor is there any mightiness in our self-manufactured idols. On the other hand, there is an enormous capacity for the power of hope to be found in our relationship with God.

Though our motives might be pure regarding how we interpret our future hope, we can still stumble over what it truly means and what it brings to our latter days.

Hope isn't a bargaining chip you can use to pressure God into giving you what you want. You can't negotiate your life with God, expecting something preferable over having desperate times of chronic suffering. The realization of hope doesn't happen when you're exclusively focusing your desires on a Cinderella future.

When we combine the Cinderella story with a confused version of our faith, we wind up with a twisted philosophy that breeds false hope. This way of thinking is inherently destructive to our faith. Moreover, false hope can quickly drain your will to get through life's difficulties. Even though you've built your life on a solid rock, this doesn't mean you're immune from the lethal doses of how false hope can reappear to quickly destroy your mind, emotions, and will.

If false hope were to look at itself in a mirror, it would see broken promises staring right back. This kind of distorted thinking underscores the impotence of human-made power, which tries to challenge the real strength of God's powerful grace. False hope delivers nothing to you except heartache and disappointment. On the other hand, God's promises will renew your strength and save those who are crushed in spirit.

On the other hand, pure hope primarily depends on God's character and nature. Who, and not what, becomes the object of hope. When you place the fullness of your humanity in Christ, you're putting all of who you are, including the brokenness, shame, and insufficiencies, back into the place where it originates—back to its source to resupply your walk of faith with restorative power. It is by Christ and through Christ alone that all real hope sustains endlessly. It does not disappoint us, even in our times of horrendous trials and tribulations.

How can God's hope let us down?

It truly can't since we have an unbreakable union with God. Although we grow weary at times, we can firmly count on an inspiration of hope further down our rocky road of life. It inspires us to endure, have self-control and patience, and become mighty because of God's nature. Our character grows within our new identity of faith, freely giving us the eternal future that God promised.

From God, hope begets hope. When your inner cup contains even a drop of hope about your circumstances, you'll experience the real-life possibilities of joy rushing into your life. Though you might feel remotely distant from where you want to be, hope returns your joy and will inspire your next steps of faith.

Don't let an edition of imperfect hope (world philosophies mixed with God's wisdom) falsely imitate God's real hope. As an alternative, turn your spiritual eyes to Him to glean the benefits of your belief. Through your faith in Him, God promises to disclose the narrative of your eternal life to you, personally, through His Word, and with absolute certainty.

Consider these encouraging thoughts about saving hope as being awakened to the truth of God. When you seem to have nothing to hope for, dare to put all of it in everything about who God is. He is the source of your confidence in faith. You can be sure that your restorative hope consists of God's love and His inexhaustible mercy.

FAITH FOR THE LONG HAUL

Do you remember when you had your salvation experience? Perhaps you carry memories similar to this life-changing account in this section.

The very idea that your sin was washed away by the blood of Jesus gave you eternal hope. Not only did your newfound conviction brightly shine within you and all around you, but so did God's love. You felt an abundance of hope and love and unspeakable peace within your cleansed heart as never before.

The heavy weight of sin and the complicated stresses of this world completely evaporated from your soul, lifting a toxic burden you had carried for years. Your salvation was a once-in-a-lifetime experience where you died to your old self and became a new person in Christ. Undoubtedly, you'll remember this rebirth for the rest of your days.

You felt free beyond words, ready to look at your life through eternal optics. You wanted to take advantage of your second chance at living your life to its fullest. Regardless of any obstacles you were facing, you were firmly determined to walk with the same love you had generously received from God.

Light was shining everywhere. You realized that God isn't part of darkness or evil. Instead, He is a brilliant light, illuminating and transforming everything He touches into something lovely and beautiful. Your conversion from old to new brought a sense of heaven into your life. Everything about your fresh-start reality carried superior value when salvation turned your former thoughts into an emerging new growth of love.

So, what about faith?

All of us are novices when walking out our faith after being reborn in the Spirit. Like babies exiting the birth canal, we're unfamiliar with what it means to be entirely human. When asked to walk out our faith, the reality is that we do not even know how to crawl yet.

Though we've experienced this new freedom in Christ through salvation, and we're initially charged emotionally with love toward God, in all likelihood, we have not even considered what it means to reach spiritual maturity.

Learning to crawl, then walk, then run, both fast-paced and marathon-like, are legitimate steps toward becoming mature in our faith. But stepping out from our former lives into His usually takes on fierce and challenging trials that will happen over several years before we really understand what it means to depend on God entirely.

At the start, we take our salvation experience very seriously as we posture ourselves for evolving change. We're highly motivated to learn various spiritual disciplines. We read and carefully study the Word. Then we progress in our faith as we acquire a developing yet deepening relationship with God through sincere prayer.

We learn how to worship God through an assortment of musical genres. We watch for those who are pillars of integrity as we attempt to imitate the best practices of their walk. Then we travel further into our sacrificial work for God. We might get heavily involved with various ministry programs as we try to discover our gifts. Moreover, we step into tithing concepts and continually discern how to give more money as prompted by our top pastoral leaders.

Over the years, our wobbly steps of faith eventually grow into fast-paced strides toward God. We try to do whatever it takes to be right with Him and remain in His good graces. On the other hand, our impression of an acceleration of spiritual growth does not prevent unwanted trials and tribulations from entering our lives.

When painful suffering pours into us, what do we do next?

Why didn't our righteous efforts prevent our unexpected disasters?

Of course, the tendency is to do whatever we've learned throughout our faith journey and implement the best spiritual practices against horrific suffering. But when the searing pain courses through our frayed nerves and refuses to comply with our prayer requests, we find ourselves reevaluating every aspect of our doctrinal beliefs, even back to when we took our first baby steps of faith.

We may even start to doubt whether we got it all wrong about conforming to the Christian religion, thinking we may have invested our lives in a fraudulent scheme.

Though it appears we are moving backward in our walk, sometimes the truth is that we might propel forwards because we've shed an extra load of unnecessary religious habits from our lives. Instead, the power of God, which is part of His mighty grace, arises in our weakest areas.

No one would choose to experience a life of chronic suffering. However, long-term fiery pain has a way of stripping some of the superficial fluff from our renditions of religiosity. It thoroughly tests the strength of the foundation of what we actually believe.

In the end, it's the smaller steps of power-packed faith that lead to massive transformation. It's learning that it's not what you're doing in your faith that determines your spirituality but the origin of what you're doing.

CHRIST ALONE

As much as we desire to have a constant light directed into our lives during our faith walk, this aspiration is historically unrealistic.

As you're dying to yourself while going through a gloomy season, you seldom see any light to guide you out of your painful miseries. You search for God, and many times, you do not find Him. You try to listen for His voice, and you end up sitting in total silence. You try to unlearn the things about your faith that are either useless or unnecessary about your new life with God. You will also have to give up the ideology often taught in the American Church that God is our self-help guide. Sometimes, and understandably, when you give up the unnecessary parts of your faith, you'll become more confused than ever.

Even as saintly as Mother Teresa was, she still experienced years of being in dark places when all she felt of God was His absence. Nevertheless, Mother Teresa persevered in faith, reframing her thoughts from herself and onto the bigger picture of life. Her loneliness represented how she could connect with Christ's personhood, for what He might have felt toward God when believing He had been forsaken by Him while being tortured and then while hanging on the cross.

Though we want our lives guided by God's truth, our lost ways, even in the darkest valleys, are not typically caused by the errors of our faith. Our faith becomes tangled because of our cowardice to overcome the fears we have to face in the stressful intersections of our lives.

As a result, we manufacture all kinds of idols in our hearts to combat our fears. We tightly hold on to the worldly gods that bring us sufficient comfort, give us a sense of power, and make overall intellectual sense along with our beliefs. We end up mixing everything we perceive as good from the world into God's grace.

Instead of persevering in our purest form of faith, we tend to act like the Israelites wandering in the desert. We get sidetracked by other gods. So often, the other gods seem innocent enough and compatible with our brokenness. Even our thoughts can become idols when we listen to the voices that whisper, "Nobody understands what you're going through"; "No one understands how bad your pain causes your misery"; and "You are the one living person who doesn't deserve this type of suffering."

The Lord's heart breaks when we seek things that are so temporal over what He has planned for our eternal inheritance.

Even when we're faithless, the truth reminds us that God remains faithful. God is faithful to us because He cannot stop being committed to Himself. He put His plan of reconciliation into motion for our beginning, our middle, and our end. He alone is the plan, living inside everyone who believes in Him. We do not have the power nor the wisdom to rewrite His plan to fit into our life agendas, no matter how hard we try.

Often, the plot has a storyline that we might not have asked for or strongly hesitated to receive. Yet from the beginning of time and throughout our modern age, our faith boils down to this truth about spirituality: what the Lord desires from us is an openly honest heart that fully returns to Him.

When there doesn't appear to be a light to follow, your only guidance might be having faith in the brighter days ahead. When you follow that belief down a long-winding dark road, you'll discover a flicker of dull light that emerges from within you. It becomes brighter the closer you get to God. Then when you return to Him, you're going to discover a new revelation about your relationship with Him. That darkness you experience is not dark to God whatsoever.

Even in our humanness and with all of our imperfections, and as we draw nearer to God, He loves us far more than we love Him. We often fool ourselves into thinking we can automatically muster up more passionate love toward Him at this point, but this isn't true. Simply put, we cannot out love God. We are considered the highest among all His creation, and He loves us the most.

Return to Him and lay down your pain again this very day. Do not linger in the war of your mind against fiery arrows of doubt. Allow the hope of God to inspire your soul to keep steadfast on the journey. Embrace the love of God to fortify your steps of faith.

When your problems are too big to handle, your far-more critical response is to let nothing about your seemingly dreary circumstances overshadow the Spirit of Jesus Christ, who resides within your heart.

He is the light where our attention needs to shift because in Him, we can see the light to walk out our faith victoriously during this lifelong pilgrimage.

NEW BEGINNINGS

DESPITE THE CHANGING DYNAMICS of our chronic suffering, the actual challenge that we face begins with us. No one else is to blame for our life of chronic pain. Nor do the reasons we suffer, whether right or wrong or how we got here, justify our hesitation to take full accountability for our circumstances.

We are not alone. God lives within us through His Holy Spirit. This fact remains. The Holy Spirit's groaning patterns within us do not mean that the Spirit of God is always grieving for us during our life of suffering. On the contrary, the Spirit Himself, who is intricately part of our inner transformation, "intercedes for us with groans that are too deep for words" (Romans 8:26b).

His intercession is firmly based on the will of God rather than our emotional interpretations regarding our pain afflictions.

The way the Holy Spirit communicates with God, and then with us, is far beyond what we can possibly understand.

We know His words work intensely on our behalf. He offers comfort, personal conviction, and guidance as we try to wrap our heads around our painful trials that represent an incredible journey of change.

Here, God's desires involve creativity, especially when we're becoming that new person who embodies the image of Christ. Because God's nature is infinite, His thumbprint on creativity is continually revealing His genius about the mysteries of what lies ahead for all of us tomorrow.

Where we get stuck is within ourselves! Tormented by pain and wracked with doubt, we are reluctant to trust God and follow the path He has laid out for us. We all deal with endless battles of uncertainty about our present and future lives. None of us wants to travel down the entire road of chronic pain until its unpromising end. We would rather have a hopeful course correction in our lives. We'd rather change direction onto the new highway of living so that we don't stay on our broken-down paths that reach the place of complete despair.

We know that our minds can become battlefields where faith, doubt, and contradictory beliefs wage war. When our logical decision-making processes bow down to fear, we can grow too afraid to step forward in faith.

As you make this journey of change, consider that you need to renew your mind always in the Spirit. You'll need the Spirit's life-giving connection to stand courageously against fear. What's more is that His Spirit can do abundantly far more than what you ask or think. This power openly lives inside you, ready to work on your behalf whenever asked, or remarkably, even when you don't ask for specific transformative steps to happen. The Holy Spirit continues the process of inner transformation, regardless.

Before you step onward into your new beginnings, do not allow all of your reasoning to narrow your scope about faith or limit the new person you're becoming day by day. It's time to seize the moment and realize that each day brings unique occasions that offer you unprecedented opportunities to experience unfamiliar but fresh aspects of life, in which you can share in the legitimate purposes of God.

CAN YOU GET STARTED?

The goal for chronic pain sufferers is to become NEW on the inside. However, we cannot trust that our physical bodies and mental traumas will respond favorably to further cutting-edge treatments of modern medicine, or for that matter, to any increasingly popular alternative.

We understand that some physical laws within our bodies do not bend to our pain-free desires. God has already given us extraordinary healing capabilities as notably demonstrated by how our bodies respond against viruses, cuts and scrapes, and all means of illness and disease. Clearly, our bodies carry an innate and independent healing quality without the assistance of human intervention.

But when our physiological responses lack the power to heal our injuries, even with terrific medicine and faithful prayer, we have to look deeper to assess the meaning behind our painful afflictions.

Temporary relief does not adequately answer the question as to why we suffer, nor does dispensing short-term improvement tame the wild beast of chronic pain. We've lived with this pain for years and are already acquainted with the clinical phases of grief several times over. When we've reached the end of the road of traditional care, then we tend to revert to lesser techniques to nurse our chronic wounds, such as psychological denial, promising potions or drinks, additional drugs, and half-hearted prayers.

Regardless of what medical technology experts suggest, the results we experience from treatments usually remain similar to our previous therapeutic encounters, falling short of providing the realities of complete pain relief.

When you've become a veteran of chronic suffering, you begin to connect the dots between your broken bodies and your troubled souls. Your physical injuries rebel and do not follow the typical neural pathways to function accordingly to your pain cycle. The brain-to-body connection is chaotically obscured, leading to various kinds of wrongful transmissions.

Your neural responses wildly express themselves with varying degrees of agonizing discomfort throughout your body. You'll often notice that new pains show up in different areas separate from your original pain source.

You do not want to allow your spirit to become infected by the same out-of-control pain responses that your body expresses.

Realistically, you do not possess the ability to separate your physical pain from your spirit. This assignment is not yours to handle, and it happens during your walk of faith.

The enemy tries to win the fight, whether it's with resistive forces, darkness, or evil, even before you can begin.

At the starting line, your mind confronts several mammoth-size fears about your constant pain. You try to consolidate your thoughts to make the right decisions against seemingly unbeatable odds.

All the while, the enemy tries to convince us that our place of darkness is darker than the darkest color imaginable and that our walk of faith can't help us climb the tallest mountains of our life's journey. These double-minded doubts do not stop, as these negative thoughts try to pull us in to two separate directions. We become more disillusioned as we see the impossibilities as way too big to overcome by our spiritual beliefs or our human capabilities.

The combination of what we hear and how we see things directly impacts our confidence of faith and our ability to get started on an arduous walk to become God's new creation. Just as significantly, if we become complacent with our faith and submit to our giant-size fears, then this will undoubtedly thwart our search to live abundantly through our pain.

Even though our bodies may be a source of continual suffering, that doesn't mean our inner beings must be condemned to a similar agony.

REACH THE POINT OF ENDURANCE

Perspective is powerful.

Chronic pain tries to keep our mindsets within that place of lukewarmness. It would be much easier to remain frigidly cold and not start our walk on the path of new beginnings. But that's not what God asks us to do. A lukewarm faith burns cool, but God wants us inflamed with passion toward becoming that new person in Christ where we can share our comforting lessons about suffering with everyone else who suffers.

To overcome the world and all of our atrocious problems, we can start with one powerful tool at our disposal. We are not required to create any supernatural weapons of warfare, nor are we expected to leap tall buildings in a single bound. Instead, we are called to overcome this world by our faith. That's right—by our faith.

Knowing the power behind our faith, our enemy tries to crush our spirits and obliterate our hopes and beliefs about wholeness and God's grace.

You are made whole through your rebirth in the Spirit. But this doesn't mean that wholeness promises pain-free healing. The enemy knows your vulnerabilities quite well about this topic and how it shapes your identity in Christ. You do not have to surrender to the death rattle of hopelessness shaken by the enemy within your mind. Rather, look beyond your small world of pain and enter into your vast universe of new life that you've received by faith.

Restored wholeness through Christ will become your hallmark, even if pain or the enemy tries to persuade you otherwise. In essence, wholeness is of deeper significance in your chronic suffering.

But we can't relax in our restoration because the enemy relentlessly tries to discourage a consistent, long-lasting faith. However, when we develop our walk with perseverance, our faith reassures us that we will feel perfect. In other words, perfect means ideally; it's as good as it gets. We can become complete in our transformation even though our bodies still show evidence of physical brokenness.

The ability to undergo painful trials through our faith in Christ turns our suffering into transformation. Longer-lasting endurance represents spiritual maturity in which God clearly states that He will provide for all of our needs, though our bodies and souls continually experience long-suffering. Our enemy does not want us to reach this point in our journey of enduring faith. In our perseverance, we will lack for nothing in our lifetime battles against trials and chronic suffering.

When you reach the end of yourself, you will probably refrain from entirely trusting yourself to carry the sticky encumbrances of this world. Because of pain alone, you'll have to unpack these heavy burdens that you've been carrying for too many years.

Once your weightiness dissipates from your former life, then you can begin to trust God for your new life to come. If you choose this path of moving straightforward to God, you'll start to learn how to fully trust in Him, the author of life who raises those of faith from the deadening darkness.

Do you want to quit your walk of faith at the starting line?

Or do you want to endure, regardless of your chronic suffering, toward the finishing line from your new beginnings?

THE IMPORTANCE OF YOUR RESPONSE

Everyone has pain. The question is, how will you address it?

It's optimal to mentally get in front of your pain rather than remaining behind and underneath it. You are called to be the head and not the tail over making important decisions regarding your life. When assuming the leadership role, you have to do it with fortified courage, as there are many hurdles to overcome along the way.

As a prime example of how to get in front of unspeakable hardships, study Guido, the father character in the 1997 Italian comedy-drama film, *Life is Beautiful*. Guido is the father of a Jewish family living in Italy at the time when Hitler's Nazi troops take over. The family is divided with the mother going to one death camp while Guido and their five-year-old son, Giosue, are sent to another concentration camp.

Immediately, all human freedoms are violently taken away from them. Nothing but the clothes on their backs remain from their former lives. They have no books or photos to enjoy, only the horrors of their rat-infested death camp.

Father and son have every excuse to give in to hopelessness and despair. Still, Guido is determined to shield his son from the horrors surrounding them by injecting humor and optimism into the bleakest of circumstances. He convinces his son that they are part of an elaborate game and that Giosue will earn points by playing hide-and-seek and engaging in other fun activities. Dad promises that when the boy earns 1,000 points, he will win a tank.

Guido's private games help give his son hope and enjoyable moments of fun and laughter amid the despair, starvation, death, and brutal humiliation of their captivity. The little boy has a smile on his face throughout the whole ordeal.

In the end, the camp is liberated. Sadly, Guido didn't survive, but Giosue does, despite the awful atrocities of war. An Allied soldier arrives and even gives Giosue a ride on his tank. Then the story concludes with Giosue eventually being reunited with his mother.

Importantly, Giosue learns valuable lessons about how to be free in your soul, even when the outside world is frighteningly horrible. These are the same lessons we can apply to our walk of faith when hope doesn't seem possible.

Life has its despairing challenges, and one of chronic suffering is nothing for which anyone would sign up. It can feel as if you're living within a quarantine concentration camp. You're continually confronting the sobering aspects of life and death that awaken you to the value of what life means.

The good news is this: you can put a different lens on your inner eyes to see your circumstances in another way, just like Guido and Giosue did.

Hopefully, you can be reminded through your insight that you are here in your earthly tent in this mortal body for a brief moment. Perhaps you are motivated to respond to your chronic suffering with renewed inspiration. It is hoped that you reach the point of laughing at the days ahead with joy that comes from your faith.

Importantly, how you respond to your new beginnings will determine the path for where you are heading. You can choose either further captivity or freedom.

Wouldn't it be great to stand in liberty, knowing that your spirit cannot be taken from you, even in dire, painful circumstances?

Your pain may not go away, but again, you can see it through a new spiritual lens and become an overcomer through how you see yourself in faith.

Your body may be held captive, but your response to your painful captivity can set you free. And this freedom will go with you by faith throughout eternity.

LIVING ABUNDANTLY

WHERE DO WE START our new beginnings in this world?

If God's ways exist in the oceans' deep waters, who can find His footprints on top of the white-capped waves? This question transcends and absolutely boggles the human mind. But when it comes to the seemingly unbelievable, all things are possible with the Spirit of God.

Doesn't our second chance at life start with following Him, whose ways are much higher than ours and whose thoughts can straighten our crooked lives?

He already knows the outcome of our faith-walk through our painful trials. So, why not loyally follow Him to start our lives on a new course?

TRUTH PROVIDES MEDICINE FOR YOUR SOUL

We cannot fix everything in our lives before we go forth toward abundant living. The starting point to deal with chronic suffering begins as we choose to change our focus to having a present mindset.

To combat the competing questions that run through our minds and try to prevent our transformation, we must have alternative thoughts that bring us life.

Sure, there are extraordinary speakers and motivational coaches who offer some nuggets of inspiration. Usually, though, their advice helps to place a temporary bandage over our painful wounds. The finest of self-help instruction seems to offer short-term bursts of motivational excitement as well as provisional hope. But for us who live with chronic pain and other debilitating conditions, we need more than an hour or two of inspirational fireworks to achieve long-lasting change.

We require words of medicine that will dispense truth into our souls. We need to experience more prolonged bouts of freedom to allow our curiosities to see the colorful perspectives about life. We're tired of the black-and-white scenarios that make up our outlooks toward a lifestyle of chronic suffering.

We can see the greener grass of hope, and then the next second, our worldview seems dark and gloomy, crushing the air out of our chests. This dithering of our thoughtful wishes takes our breath away, and not in the right way. We're usually dealing with significant bouts of depression and anxiety, which typically accompany long-term physical and mental conditions.

It's only when we realize that we can't fix ourselves perfectly that we become open to unfamiliar or initially dismissed perspectives toward pain relief and the possibility of healing.

GAINING GOD'S PERSPECTIVE

Almost everything in life has different perspectives to consider, and there are as many translations about chronic suffering as there are with anything else.

Where do you find these versions of truth that will open your eyes to more effective ways of living with chronic pain?

There are two reliable sources that you might want to consider. First, God's Word provides powerful truth that changes how you think, what you value, and how you change your behaviors. The Word helps you focus on your present circumstances and offers you an infinite future of life-changing doorways that you can freely walk through by God's special invitation. New things, new ways, abundant love, and numerous blessings await your steps of faith.

Chronic suffering is not the victor over God's love for your life. Nor is your life doomed to defeat in this world before passing into paradise after death. The Word provides the armaments to fight your battles against the real enemy of your life. Though pain seems to be your enemy, it isn't. Suffering strengthens your inner person to recognize who the real enemy is. Through devastating trials, your enduring faith gives you the strength to stand firm when your life's intense battles are way above your abilities.

Second, consider the most recognizable symbol about life and death integrated within our human culture for the past 2,000-plus years—the figure of the cross. For Jesus, the cross meant that the world's entire weight and every sin of man had to be carried by Him in a painfully gruesome death. He knew everything about our lives, including our painful afflictions and disappointments. Because of His love for us, He still decided to bear our offenses on that splintery wooden cross.

For us, we have a less-painful reminder when we observe the meaning behind the fullness of the cross. Staring at it brings us to a place of repentance so that we don't have to carry our sin's weight. It's where we intersect with the God of the universes who connected with us first. It is where the divine and humanity touch through suffering to bring about full redemption for humankind. We cannot redeem ourselves. Likewise, on the cross, we can practically see our limitations to cure our chronic afflictions miraculously.

The Living Word and the cross certainly offer credible translations of suffering and redemptive healing for all humanity.

TRUST IN HOW GOD SEES YOU

In essence, living abundantly occurs when we actually "live-out" our faith, regardless of the potential pitfalls we might face. An abundant lifestyle significantly pulls our focus off our pains, even temporarily, and places it on an inspired vision for better living.

No matter the road you choose to achieve this goal of abundance, you'll most likely discover that nearly all roads lead to one conclusion—heading directly to a sanctified life, one that solidifies your faith into eternal practices. It's the kind that underscores that you've been set apart for something very unique. It emphasizes a purposeful life guided by the Holy Spirit to produce good works, regardless of how you view your own capacity to accomplish these assignments.

Before you can see yourself as light, you must believe how God sees who you are, even in the worst times of your suffering. It's not how you see yourself emotionally, especially if you're digesting negative thoughts about your heavy-hearted circumstances. Instead, how God sees you is the truth of what your entire being will eventually personify.

When you see yourself in His light, then you'll embark on the reconciliation of your long-term hurts and find yourself aligning with the truth of God's plan for you.

When we know God as He truly is, then we'll introspectively discover who we actually are in the scheme of our relationship with Him. Once we know ourselves more clearly, we can proceed joyfully onto the dance floor of life. As we attempt to follow God's intricate rhythms and learn His beautiful dance steps, we will know more comprehensibly what it means to live more abundantly.

COMMIT TO INNER CHANGE

For transformation to happen in your life, you must make a rock-solid decision to commit yourself entirely to making these mighty changes.

Whether we have broken-down bodies or badly wounded hearts, full commitment requires every part of us to participate in the process of transformation.

Set aside the weight about what hasn't been accomplished due to your long-term suffering, and instead, totally commit your broken body to God as you begin your steps of restoration. In effect, this opens the doors to your purpose—to offer your entire body to God as your ongoing spiritual worship.

As you worship God with your whole being, this adoration of Him strips away your false self that tends to build upon your recurring pain. You'll discover that your worship of God in songs of adoration and with every working element of your life uncovers the realness of who you are. When you see yourself as you really are, it seems as if your sense of hope becomes replenished.

Your empty cup now fills up to the brim with hope. Like a domino effect, your hope supplies more confidence in your life. Step by step, your new hope brings encouragement to your enduring faith. Before you know it, your life thirsts for your time of worship with God. It has become your sacred place for you and Him, a watering hole of sharing in your afflictions and gleaning comfort through His presence.

While it's natural to assume that you are doing all the work to worship God by presenting your body to Him, this belief is not entirely true.

You're not doing all the work. God participates as well.

Who is God in these instances of our spiritual worship to Him?

Well, God is not the highest version of your sense of self. Though you unpack the false layers of who you are during this time with Him, God remains as He is—our Creator and our Savior and our only God.

He already knows the number of hairs on your head at any given moment. The Spirit of His worship doesn't demand petitions or remorsefulness. Instead, God delights in your discovery of having adoration for Him. These hidden treasures of love are discovered by deeper faith that comes from suffering. No longer does your sense of brokenness need to usurp the evolving love that's growing toward Him. In effect, you must not make your painful problems bigger than Him.

How we perceive truthfulness on the surface does not necessarily expose the actual truth of what exists. For example, God's depth of knowledge presents beauty when we see only burnt ashes. That's why He invites us to worship Him, not partially but thoroughly with our whole bodies to see more of His nature and why we experience horrendous pain as part of our whole-person growth.

Because of His eternal promises of redemption, He encourages us to become partakers of His divine nature. Christ wants us to touch His robe to receive the power of healing, though oftentimes, many of us do not experience a complete absence of pain. Yet God desires us to see the deeper parts of healing, in which wholeness inspires our growing love for Him.

Abundant living happens when you commit to begin your remarkable change. And vitally important, you must maintain your responsibility to stay on the path of transformation. You also must play your role in experiencing the life-giving benefits of your upcoming changes.

When you start to see yourself anew, your dedication to this vision will bring some highly positive results.

PRACTICE HOLY LIVING

What does it mean to present your body as a living sacrifice to God?

Will this act lead to your healing?

Our bodies do not refer exclusively to our outer shells of flesh and bones. Instead, our bodies also incorporate every part of who we are that makes up our whole person, such as our minds, emotions, and will. When we present our bodies as living sacrifices, we surrender our whole being (how we live) to God under His direction.

Giving our entire lives to God is a deliberate choice we can voluntarily make when we worship Him. We do not have to have healthy bodies to offer ourselves to God for His approval. By His grace, we can come as we are, whether weak, pain-ridden, hungry, or thirsty, to enter into a time of contemplative worship.

Especially for us who suffer from painful afflictions, our frail bodies and lifestyle vulnerabilities are all we can give to God. Our worship times desire to have the platforms of reverence and connection, two components that are sorely missing from our everyday lives.

As we're confronted daily with the more profound questions about life and death and continuously feel whittled away by the physical realities of ongoing pain and fatigue, we look forward to bringing all our daunting thoughts to God. We know that His eyes are not blind to His weakest worshippers. We can give our entire beings, whether painfully expressive or not, to God by submitting our all in all to Him.

When you continually choose to provide your whole person to God, in a sense, you're undergoing the kind of transformation that slowly changes you into the image of Christ, who was the perfect embodiment of holy living.

For some, this process doesn't feel like transformation. There is no quick-fix evidence associated with deliberately rededicating your life to God. But if you undergo the complete process of inner change, this slow-moving transformation significantly changes who you are from the inside out.

Your mind begins to resemble the truth found in Scripture. Your emotions start to follow the truth about who you are instead of aligning yourself with the screeching sounds of pain that battle for your attention. Your thoughts navigate between God and suffering. But when you get a temporary break from the pain, then your concentration becomes keenly aware of the unique relationship that's developing between Christ and you.

Dedicating yourself to God is not a one-time process but a moment-by-moment commitment. You must dig deep to change your attitudes about yourself, God, and the environment around you, including others who may have caused you harm unintentionally. When you surrender yourself to God, you vulnerably open your life in spirit and truth *only* to Him.

No comparisons allowed. You're not in competition with anyone else, including other healthy and seemingly prosperous believers, to prove your worth to God.

Your act of service starts with your private confessions to God. It's like you're an onion being peeled through several layers of trauma. God wants your honest and sincere sacrifice unto Him. He desires to transform your life's loathsome difficulties into a holy fragrance, which becomes pleasing to everyone who breathes life through their spiritual senses.

In a nutshell, suffering grows you deeper spiritually. Making a long-term commitment to give your whole being to God leads you into a beautiful transformation of both your character and your physical body.

Holy living is living abundantly.

So, why not be part of something greater than you ever imagined?

DON'T STOP

STRAIGHT PATHS are the most efficient ways to get where you want to go and accomplish what you want to do. But sometimes, taking the straight paths can seem rather monotonous and boring.

In today's fast-moving, instant-gratification-seeking world, we're no longer satisfied with quick and speedy answers to our complicated situations. We want to take it up a notch with faster answers and immediate results to rid us of our pains and spare us from getting hurt by the sharp objects of life.

For those who chronically suffer, the quick-fix answers and the miraculous solutions rarely occur as evidenced by the millions who continue to bear the brunt of a pain-ridden lifestyle.

Plain and simple: there are no shortcuts about what it takes to live abundantly through our chronic sufferings.

Chronic pain not only affects our physical bodies adversely, but its destructive nature also attaches itself to every part of our lives, including our souls, our work, our purpose, our families, our hobbies, our rest, our communities, and our churches. There is not one area of our lives that's immune from the damage caused by pain's stinging tentacles.

The strangling arms of pain limit what chronic sufferers can do. We are unable to multitask. We're practically incapable of keeping to rigid schedules, whether for personal reasons or medical appointments. We regularly offer flimsy excuses to justify our weakness, lateness, or absence from meetings or gatherings.

Suffering divides the innermost parts of who we are. We risk confusing or offending our closest friends and family because we can't meet their most basic expectations. For instance, whenever we're invited to a family event or social gathering, we know that the pain we're going to incur from the outing will far outweigh the value of the whole social experience. Our complicit response to chronic suffering encourages isolation and dislocates us from the dynamics of our surrounding communities.

As everything about our lives seems to swirl out of control, we fail in our attempts to be active and disciplined. We find we must occasionally slow down momentarily before responding to the next episode of grueling adversities.

Chaos and buzzing noises throughout our bodies and minds remind us how raw our nerves and emotions are. As our inner world seems as if it's in a perpetual state of disarray, our outer world grows equally chaotic. We instinctively realize that it's going to take a hard fight on our part to fit into life again.

We feel disabled when compared to those who live healthy lives. We lack the energy and the physical stamina to keep up with them as this fast-paced world continues to spin rapidly. Our diseases and illnesses have shattered the organized patterns of our existence, demolishing any hope that we may have left to regain some momentum to live abundantly.

MAKING YOUR PATH STRAIGHT

Even while suffering, there is hope. At times, our yearnings for relief are misplaced in the wrong things or unsuitable places. We can't expect our hope to rescue us from our sufferings instantaneously. Even the spiritually mature can get sidetracked, venturing off the straight path to God and going astray from the call of holy living.

Instead of desperately falling for anything that looks promising, we need to step back from the chaos, pause, and breathe for a moment.

Don't fill your thoughts with shame or regret about back-sliding from your pursuits of abundant living. When the negative thoughts press into you, simply stand against them. You do not have to make any quick and foolish choices about getting rid of negativity or the chaos of pain.

Rather, concentrate on breathing in and then breathing out. Turn your breathing time into a contemplative meditation session.

Allow yourself to mentally and physically inhale and exhale the broken rhythms of your life. There is no need to be embarrassed by the starts and stops in your breathing patterns due to your ailing body and anxious thoughts.

Sharply focus on receiving God's forgiveness when breathing in. Then as you breathe out from way down deep, release His mercy to others around you. This simple exercise will become an act of forgiveness toward your painful suffering.

When God's forgiveness becomes part of your rhythms, you'll discover that your paths will straighten out because of the grace of Jesus Christ.

Continue to surrender all the parts of your life to God. Step into each area by faith and boldly confront the collateral damage. You will have features that won't be repairable. And that's okay. God doesn't want you to focus all your energy on restoring the old, broken pieces. Instead, He encourages you to trust in Him to give you new experiences that will replace and possibly transcend what you're accustomed to.

Courageously walk through the fire of your suffering to the other side of freedom. Your purification will benefit your spiritual growth, and it will propel you straightforward into the comforting arms of Jesus Christ.

DISCIPLINE FUELS YOUR SPIRITUAL GROWTH

Next, learn to focus on your present mindset. Patiently give yourself a mental break when you experience some bumps in the road.

There is no place where your body, purpose, or light will explore without your mind first envisioning this expedition.

Imagine that the Holy Spirit operates like the wind. His ideas might seem fleeting. If your brain is buzzing and chaotic, you might dismiss God speaking through His Holy Spirit to you. It would help if you slowed down your life to gain the vision and wisdom for what the Holy Spirit is generously trying to hand you. When all is said and done, He is actively trying to get your attention to strengthen your building faith.

Keep focused on renewing your mindset and not conform to the ways of this world. In all likelihood, your chronic pain will not let you do what you once did. Discover new interests and ways of reshaping your finances, adopting essentialism, and finding those things and people who genuinely bring you joy.

Allow God to reorganize your thoughts amid the disastrous areas of your mind. Allow Him to rewire your thinking by the Holy Spirit's promptings and through the truth of His Word that you can follow by faith.

To follow Him and allow new things to shape your walk of faith, you must arm yourself with an iron hand of discipline. You must fight hard every day to persevere during your battles against suffering. To see transforming changes occur, you must not give in to discouragement or despair or self-indulgence. If you apply hard work and discipline to your doubts and fears, you will help fuel your spiritual growth, even amid your weariness.

If you sense your life is far from abundant, don't give up. If you happen to go backward again due to unforeseeable circumstances, don't be discouraged. No matter how you feel, you still have control over your attitudes.

Your life's enemy is not your troubling circumstances or your nagging pain or your desperate thoughts, but it is the evil one who opposes you. The meaning behind your fiery tests will be determined by how you respond to your ongoing trials.

PRACTICE NEW HABITS

When your suffering presses you to swear at your painful afflictions and hardships, try going against those human reflexes. Instead of swearing, sing a new song of adoration to God.

It can be challenging to fine-tune your voice when trying to wipe away the tears. But once you gain your composure, you'll find that though your songs' lyrics ring familiar, the actual words gain power as you sing them through your painful times.

If you are unable to sing, then try to pray. If the words have escaped your mind, then learn how to listen to the Holy Spirit. He will guide you into praying. Seek out silence if you do not know how to sing or pray.

This state of quietness and stillness provides opportunities to reenergize your contemplative thoughts. Or you can read some Scripture verses and pray these words right back into your soul. You'll be amazed at how much the truth of the Word spoon-feeds healing into your being.

Through your practice of discipline, you're now a partner with the Holy Spirit on this incredible journey. God's grace will provide His power to see you through any of your inadequacies and weaknesses. The godly and uplifting things you can't see will become visible to your eyes through the hard work of your disciplined hand.

Continue to believe without ceasing. You'll find that your hope in God will be restored as long as you keep believing in Him for your life's sovereign direction. Let God remove the enormous obstacles from your rocky road and watch as He gives you your heart's desires.

It's uncanny how God delivers us from our rabbit holes of anguish and places us onto the higher ground to start all over again.

You'll discover that God's fundamental purpose is not to "fix" every problem in your life but to give you a new heart, a new mind, and a new resurrected body for your ultimate destination.

If you've experienced chronic suffering for decades, your purpose will likely be found in your pain. Much of your purpose shifts from problem-solving and climbing the ladder of success to becoming a preparer of God's Kingdom. This world's ambitions will no longer easily tempt you away from God's path as you are increasingly able to set your sights on spiritual purposes that will grow your gifts, regardless of your chronically battered condition.

Growth is possible though you're painfully tired. As the days pass, and you don't seem to have accomplished anything in your life, you'll eventually look back at your suffering days and realize that God was doing His reconstructive work within your inward life without you realizing it at the time.

When you begin to recognize and embrace the growth of your inward life, you'll become more life-giving to yourself and others. What's equally beautiful is that the Holy Spirit within you is integrally part of your growth process and is beside you, in back of you, below you, and in front of your straight path to God.

THE POWER OF PRAYER

Do not underestimate the power of prayer. Though chronic pain can make your prayers seem powerless, this is not the truth about your relational connection to God. In a way, you must approach prayer like you do strict discipline. Be sober and mindful about your prayer life as you're facing ongoing battles against a formidable enemy who does not want you to succeed in your walk of faith.

As Henri Nouwen eloquently states, "Prayer is far from sweet and easy. Being the expression of our greatest love, it does not keep the pain away. Instead, it makes us suffer more since our love for God is a love for a suffering God. Our entering into God's intimacy is an entering into intimacy where all of human suffering is embraced in divine compassion."

Keep moving in faith and prayer, regardless of the speed and magnitude, and do not stop!

YOUR LIFETIME MAINTENANCE PLAN

Dedicating yourself to God doesn't require you to be perfect, just committed. Understandably, it's hard to give yourself to God when pain tries to jolt you off your center. Maintaining a commitment to God seems unrealistic when you do not get a timely reprieve from your thorny pain.

But do not complicate things by putting more expectations upon yourself than necessary to dedicate your life to Christ. You do not have to make yourself perfect. You do not have to obsess about your diet or exercise or sleeping standards, though these practical ways contribute significantly to better health and holy living.

When you put too many self-imposed disciplines on your plate, you'll eventually get tired of gorging your lifestyle with too many expectations. Likely, you'll still experience frequent episodes of pain and will probably abandon your newly designed lifestyle of commitment.

We need to wrap our heads mentally around eternal finish lines. Without a sense of these boundaries, we tend to lose the inspiring vision for our lives.

Even when it comes to your final resting place at the end of your days, you no longer need to be anxious. Rather, you can walk forward with new intentions and renewed hope.

You are no longer bound by what the world expects of you. You can change the focus of your real purpose, free from the shackles of others' expectations. You can learn to retreat during the storms of pain. No one can hold you back from entering into a silent place to get some rest. No other power can summon you away from living a transformed life until you reach the finish line.

There is no rest for your heart except in and with God. When you maintain your commitment to give your whole being to God as a living sacrifice, you're not merely visiting Him during regularly scheduled hours; you're carrying Him full time throughout all parts of your life. You're no longer alone. He's transforming every aspect of your nature for your final seasons. God inhabits you permanently. He doesn't just visit you occasionally when you act religiously pleasing to Him.

God is now abundantly part of you in every respect, here and now and forever afterward.

How much more abundant can life get?

It can't!

Don't stop!

NOTES

INTRODUCTION

- Mark 14:36
- Matthew 5:45

YOU ARE NOT ALONE

- National Center for Complementary and Integrative Health, "Defining the Prevalence of Chronic Pain in the United States," September 14, 2018, www.nccih.nih.gov.
- Matthew 13:1–23
- Deuteronomy 25:2
- Isaiah 53:10
- Mark 15:16–20

FALLING INTO THE PAIN PIT

- Author contributions: R.D. Treede, W. Rief, and A. Barke contributed equally to this topical review, "Pain," US National Library of Medicine National Institutes of Health.
- Matthew 25:31–46

WALKING WITH A LIMP

- Mark 9:23
- Philippians 3:10
- Matthew 13:1–23

WHEN YOU FEEL LIKE GIVING UP

- John 10:1–18
- Matthew 18:10–14

SANDCASTLES WASHED AWAY

- Galatians 6:8
- "Deepest Part of the Ocean: The Challenger Deep in the Mariana Trench is the deepest known location in Earth's oceans," https://geology.com/records/deepest-part-of-the-ocean.shtml.
- Hebrews 4:12
- Isaiah 7-8

- Matthew 1:22–23
- Romans 8:37
- 1 Corinthians 13
- 1 Peter 4:8

NO MORE DOUBTS

- Psalms 34:18
- Colossians 1:27
- Isaiah 40:31
- 1 John 1:5
- Psalms 119:105–107
- Exodus 32
- 2 Timothy 2:13
- Isaiah 55:6–7
- 2 Corinthians 12:9
- James 4:8
- 1 John 4:19–21
- Psalms 36:9

NEW BEGINNINGS

- Romans 8:26
- Ephesians 3:17–19
- James 1:2–4
- Revelation 3:15–21

- John 5:4
- 2 Corinthians 1:3–9
- Hebrews 12:1–3
- Deuteronomy 28:13
- Galatians 5:1

ABUNDANT LIVING

- Psalms 77:19
- Romans 6:22
- 2 Peter 1:4–10
- Psalms 33:18–22

DON'T STOP

- Hebrews 12:7–11
- Joshua 1:9
- Psalms 37:4
- Constable's Notes on Romans, 2000, pp. 130–131.
- Romans 12:1–2

Gordon & Cherise LLC

DISCLAIMERS

MEDICAL DISCLAIMER

THIS BOOK IS NOT INTENDED FOR THE PURPOSE OF PROVIDING MEDICAL ADVICE.

All information, content, and material of Gordon & Cherise LLC, including the books *Pursue Real Hope* and *Get Your Pain-filled Life on Track*, the website www.gordonandcherise.com, and the affiliated podcast programs, are for informational purposes only and not intended to serve as a substitute for the consultation, diagnosis, and/or medical treatment of a qualified physician or health-care provider.

The information supplied through or within our books or by any representative or agent of Gordon & Cherise LLC, whether by telephone, email, letter, facsimile, or other form of communication, is for informational purposes only and does not constitute medical, legal, or other professional advice. Health-related information provided through our books, website, social media, and podcasts is not a substitute for medical advice and should not be used to diagnose or treat health problems or to prescribe any medical devices or other remedies.

The information contained on this website is compiled from a variety of sources and is not considered complete. The information accessed through this website is provided *as is* and without any warranties, whether expressed or implied.

The receipt of any questions or feedback that you submit to Gordon & Cherise LLC does not create a professional relationship and does not create any privacy interests.

YOU SHOULD ALWAYS CONSULT A PHYSICIAN OR OTHER HEALTH-CARE PROVIDER OF YOUR OWN CHOICE AND CAREFULLY READ ALL PACKAGING AND OTHER INFORMATION PROVIDED BY THE MANUFACTURER OF ANY PRODUCTS OR DEVICES BEFORE USING THEM.

MEDICAL EMERGENCY

If you have a medical emergency, call your doctor or 911 immediately.

To the fullest extent permitted by law, Gordon & Cherise LLC **DISCLAIMS ALL REPRESENTATIONS AND WARRANTIES, EXPRESSED OR IMPLIED,** and makes no representation or warranty as to the reliability, accuracy, timeliness, usefulness, adequacy, or suitability of the information contained in our website, books, podcasts, and social media and does not represent and/or warrant against human or machine error, omissions, delays, interruptions, or losses, including the loss of any data.

GENERAL WEBSITE INFORMATION

The information contained in our website, www.gordonandcherise.com, is not intended to recommend the self-management of health problems or wellness. It is not intended to endorse or recommend any particular type of medical treatment. Should any reader have any health-care related questions, promptly call or consult your physician or health-care provider. No information contained in this website should be used by any reader to disregard medical and/or health-related advice or to provide a basis to delay consultation with a physician or a qualified health-care provider.

PASTORAL COUNSELING & COACHING DISCLAIMER

Counseling and ministering through book materials, website, social media, and podcasts will be provided by affiliates, including

Gordon Selley and Cherise Selley of Gordon & Cherise LLC. The counseling and rendering of lifestyle advice by Gordon & Cherise Selley are NOT licensed counseling services through the state of Colorado.

Also, Gordon Selley maintains an inactive license as a chiropractic doctor in the state of Colorado. However, Gordon Selley, DC *does not* perform any duties associated with the diagnosis and treatment of any individuals or patients due to his inactive status.

All counseling and ministering are provided in accordance with biblical principles and are not necessarily provided in adherence to any local or national psychological or psychiatric association.

No representation has been made, either expressly or implied, that biblical counseling or ministering or consulting, as conducted by the above-mentioned pastoral counselors and coaches, is accepted as customary psychological and/or psychiatric therapy within the definitional terms utilized by those professions.

In consideration for receiving any form of counseling or ministering from Gordon & Cherise LLC, the person receiving the counseling and ministering agrees to release and waive any and all claims of any kind against the business and any associated individuals, including Gordon Selley and Cherise Selley of Gordon & Cherise LLC, which may arise from, result out of, or be related to conduct or advice given.

ABOUT GORDON & CHERISE

WE ARE A COUPLE IN LOVE. Since 1996, our marriage carries an enduring hope that transcends the challenges of battling chronic pain, role reversals, blended-family issues, and owning and operating a specialized boutique-style real estate brokerage in Colorado Springs, Colorado.

Through it all, we are determined to bring energizing faith and real hope to others, regardless of their station in life.

We desire to give a voice of dignity to those who feel like they have lost their expression, to remind others that victory is on the other side of the battle that they might be facing.

We love to bring life to the human heart, and with God's grace, we desire to be part of deeply restoring beauty within peoples' lives.

Our purpose is to empower others to live the best life possible through their chronic suffering. We want to inspire people to persevere, no matter the obstacles, and to find their ultimate purpose in this present life.

Join us on this incredible journey.

Discover your new sense of health and home in a fresh and invigorating way through our platform, which delivers life-giving nourishment through the mediums of books, *The Gordon & Cherise Show* podcasts, devotionals, our website (www.gordonandcherise.com), transformational coaching, and social media (Facebook, Instagram, YouTube, Spotify and iTunes).